USING JUDGMENTS IN SECOND LANGUAGE ACQUISITION RESEARCH

Synthesizing the theory behind and methodology for conducting judgment tests, *Using Judgments in Second Language Acquisition Research* aims to clarify the issues surrounding this method and to provide best practices in its use. The text is grounded on a balanced and comprehensive background of the usage of judgment data in the past up through its present-day applications. SLA researchers and graduate students will find useful a chapter serving as a "how-to" guide for a variety of situations to conduct research using judgments, including ways to optimize task design and examples from successful studies. Lucid and practical, *Using Judgments in Second Language Acquisition Research* offers guidance on a method widely used by SLA researchers, both old and new to the field.

Patti Spinner is Associate Professor at Michigan State University. Her work focuses on the acquisition of grammar by second language learners. She has published numerous articles in journals such as *Studies in Second Language Acquisition*, *Language Learning*, *Linguistic Approaches to Bilingualism*, *Applied Linguistics*, and more.

Susan M. Gass is University Distinguished Professor at Michigan State University. She has published widely in the field of Second Language Acquisition, including the textbook *Second Language Acquisition: An Introductory Course* (Routledge), co-authored with Jennifer Behney and Luke Plonsky. She co-edits (with Alison Mackey) the Routledge series on Second Language Acquisition Research.

Second Language Acquisition Research series

Susan M. Gass and Alison Mackey, Series Editors

The *Second Language Acquisition Research* series presents and explores issues bearing directly on theory construction and/or research methods in the study of second language acquisition. Its titles (both authored and edited volumes) provide thorough and timely overviews of high-interest topics, and include key discussions of existing research findings and their implications. A special emphasis of the series is reflected in the volumes dealing with specific data collection methods or instruments. Each of these volumes addresses the kinds of research questions for which the method/instrument is best suited, offers extended description of its use, and outlines the problems associated with its use. The volumes in this series will be invaluable to students and scholars alike, and perfect for use in courses on research methodology and in individual research.

Using Judgments in Second Language Acquisition Research
Patti Spinner and Susan M. Gass

Language Aptitude
Advancing Theory, Testing, Research and Practice
Edited by Zhisheng (Edward) Wen, Peter Skehan, Adriana Biedroń, Shaofeng Li and Richard Sparks

For more information about this series, please visit:
www.routledge.com/Second-Language-Acquisition-Research-Series/book-series/LEASLARS

Of related interest:

Second Language Acquisition
An Introductory Course, Fourth Edition
Susan M. Gass with Jennifer Behney and Luke Plonsky

Second Language Research
Methodology and Design, Second Edition
Alison Mackey and Susan M. Gass

USING JUDGMENTS IN SECOND LANGUAGE ACQUISITION RESEARCH

Patti Spinner and Susan M. Gass

Routledge
Taylor & Francis Group
NEW YORK AND LONDON

First published 2019
by Routledge
52 Vanderbilt Avenue, New York, NY 10017

and by Routledge
2 Park Square, Milton Park, Abingdon, Oxon, OX14 4RN

Routledge is an imprint of the Taylor & Francis Group, an informa business

Library of Congress Cataloging-in-Publication Data
A catalog record for this book has been requested

ISBN: 978-1-138-20702-8 (hbk)
ISBN: 978-1-138-20703-5 (pbk)
ISBN: 978-1-315-46337-7 (ebk)

Typeset in Bembo
by Apex CoVantage, LLC
Printed by CPI Group (UK) Ltd, Croydon CR0 4YY

To Jon, Sam, and Joya
Patti Spinner

To Samuel, Jonah, Gabriel for whom Safta's love is at the highest end of the Likert scale
Susan M. Gass

CONTENTS

FIGURES

PREFACE

Judgments of the acceptability of grammatical constructions are a long-established source of data for linguists who seek to understand the nature of language and the limits of human language. This same elicitation technique has been widely adopted in research on second (L2) and foreign language learning. Yet, despite the frequent use of judgments, there is much that remains controversial, particularly with regard to the interpretation of judgment data and issues of elicitation and analysis.

Judgments have been and continue to be collected in many different ways and for many different purposes. This book is intended to demystify this common elicitation technique and provide guidelines for those who collect L2 data using judgments or read L2 research that employs judgments. In this book, we discuss philosophical issues, as well as more practical issues such as concerns about reliability, construct validity, appropriate participants, intervening factors (e.g., processing limitations and working memory), design, and research robustness, among others. A central goal of this book is to describe ways to design and implement studies using judgment data and to acquaint the reader with appropriate ways to interpret results from studies that utilize such data.

The book is neutral in terms of theoretical approach; we present information about judgment data use within a wide range of theoretical approaches in both second and foreign language research. We provide information about key concepts and the use of this methodology, and additionally review controversies regarding what information judgment data provide. We also present information on best and common practices in designing a study using judgments and in displaying results from such studies. In so doing, we provide numerous examples treating a range of topics. Our examples reflect a variety of perspectives, and we include illustrations from studies that reflect a range of learning contexts and differences in learning backgrounds. We also show how judgments can be used as either the sole method of elicitation or one of several elicitation techniques in a research study. Our goal is to make it easier for readers both to interpret second language studies and to construct their own studies in an informed and responsible manner.

We intend this text to serve as a guide for experienced second language researchers as well as those who are just beginning to conduct L2 research and who want to use judgments as one way of gathering data.

Patti Spinner, East Lansing, Michigan
Susan Gass, Williamston, Michigan

ACKNOWLEDGMENTS

Like many (if not most) projects, this one turned out to be longer than we expected. In the course of this journey, there are many whom we want to acknowledge and thank. First, our partners in a related project, Emma Marsden and Luke Plonsky and our graduate student (now professor), Dustin Crowther. We had already begun to work on this project when we learned of the large database on judgments that Emma and Luke were putting together. We joined forces, and together with Dustin Crowther, we published the results of that database in the journal *Second Language Research*. The resulting work is acknowledged many times over in this book.

Two reviewers provided initial feedback to us that helped us reformulate and reorganize some of our original plans. We thank them for their careful reading and excellent ideas. Luke Plonsky, throughout the process, has been of enormous assistance in sharing his ideas and expertise with us. He gave freely (and quickly) of his time. Thanks so, so much, Luke.

There were many research assistants who helped us along the way. They had many roles, including editing, finding examples, and reading for clarity. In addition to Dustin Crowther, we also acknowledge help from Jin-Soo Choi, Lizz Huntley, and Natalie Koval.

We are grateful for the support and patience from everyone at Routledge. A big thank you for having the patience and belief that we would eventually finish.

1

JUDGMENT DATA IN LINGUISTIC RESEARCH

> Linguistic intuitions became the royal way into an understanding of the competence which underlies all linguistic performance.
>
> *(Levelt, van Gent, Haans, & Meijers, 1977, p. 88)*

1.1. Introduction

Understanding what is within the confines of a grammar of a language and what is outside the grammar of a language is central to understanding the limits of human language. Householder (1973) reminds us that this concept is not new. As early as the second century of the common era, the Greek grammarian Apollonius Dyscolus conducted linguistic analysis by analyzing sentences as grammatical or ungrammatical. However, the question remains: how do we know when something is grammatical or ungrammatical beyond the spoken and/or written data provided by native speakers of a language? With a focus on second language research, this book deals with one prominent way of determining what is part of one's knowledge of language, namely, individuals' judgments of what is and what is not acceptable in any given language.

Simply put, judgment tasks require that an individual judge whether a sentence is acceptable or not. The most common way of conducting a judgment task is to present a sentence and ask whether that sentence is a possible sentence in the language being asked about. As will become clear in this book, there are many variations on this theme and many controversies surrounding the methodology.

Despite the fact that judgment tasks have been central to the linguistic scene since the early days of generative grammar, their use has been the subject of numerous discussions relating to underlying philosophical issues, as well as more practical issues such as concerns about reliability, construct validity, appropriate participants, intervening factors (such as processing limitations and working memory), design, and research robustness, among others. In this book, we intend to demystify the use of judgment tasks and to present background information about their role in furthering our understanding of native and second language grammars, as well as their role in elucidating issues surrounding the learning of second languages. A central goal of this book is to describe ways to design and implement studies using judgment data and to acquaint the reader with appropriate ways to interpret results from studies that utilize such data.

1.2. Judgment Data in Linguistics

The use of judgment data in linguistics has a long history. Early research rejected the use of anything other than production data (cf. Bloomfield, 1935). Bloomfield's arguments about linguistics as science included nonreliance on internal mental states, as they could not be verified scientifically. However, the role of judgments in linguistic work took a turn with the writings of Chomsky (1957, 1965). As Levelt et al. (1977) note, "The concept of grammaticality is a crucial one in generative linguistics since Chomsky (1957) chose it to be the very basis for defining a natural language" (p. 87). Chomsky (1965) argues early on for the importance of introspective reports when he observes that "the actual data of linguistic performance will provide much evidence for determining the correctness of hypotheses about underlying linguistic structure, along with introspective reports (by the native speaker, or the linguist who has learned the language)" (p. 18).

In Chomsky (1957), we see indirect reference to intuitions, when he states

> one way to test the adequacy of a grammar proposed for L is to determine whether or not the sequences that it generates are actually grammatical, i.e., acceptable to a native speaker. . . . For the purposes of this discussion, however, suppose that we assume intuitive knowledge of the grammatical sentences of English.
>
> *(p. 13)*

He also recognizes that using intuitional data may not be ideal:

> It is unfortunately the case that no adequate formalizable techniques are known for obtaining reliable information concerning the facts of linguistic structure. . . . There are . . . very few reliable experimental or data-processing procedures for obtaining significant information concerning the linguistic intuition of the native speaker.
>
> *(Chomsky, 1965, p. 19)*

However, the inability to gather reliable data should not be an impediment: "Even though few reliable operational procedures have been developed, the theoretical (that is, grammatical) investigation of the knowledge of the native speaker can proceed perfectly well" (Chomsky, 1965, p. 19).

Quite clearly, Chomsky's views are in direct opposition to earlier work by Bloomfield, whose statements expressed the notion that intuitional data should be removed from the realm of scientific investigation. Chomsky dismisses this challenge:

> One may ask whether the necessity for present-day linguistics to give such priority to introspective evidence and to the linguistic intuition of the native speaker excludes it from the domain of science. The answer to this essentially terminological question seems to have no bearing at all on any serious issue.
>
> *(Chomsky, 1965, p. 20)*

1.2.1. Terminology and Underlying Constructs: Grammaticality and Acceptability

Numerous terms referring to intuitional data are bandied about in the literature, and unfortunately, they are often used interchangeably even though they reflect different constructs. Primary among these terms are *grammaticality* and *acceptability*, which have different theoretical implications. We begin with Chomsky's (1965) own words about the terms *acceptability* and *grammaticality*. Many issues are incorporated in these terms, including the important difference between them and the fact that acceptability may be gradient.

> Let us use the term "acceptable" to refer to utterances that are perfectly natural and immediately comprehensible without paper-and-pencil analysis, and in no way bizarre or outlandish. Obviously, acceptability will be a matter of degree, along various dimensions. . . . The more acceptable sentences are those that are more likely to be produced, more easily understood, less clumsy, and in some sense more natural. The unacceptable sentence one would tend to avoid and replace by more acceptable variants, wherever possible, in actual discourse.
>
> The notion "acceptable" is not to be confused with "grammatical." Acceptability is a concept that belongs to the study of performance, whereas grammaticalness belongs to the study of competences. . . . Like acceptability, grammaticalness is, no doubt, a matter of degree . . . but the scales of grammaticalness and acceptability do not coincide. Grammaticalness is only one of many factors that interact to determine acceptability. Correspondingly, although one might propose various operational tests for acceptability, it is unlikely that a necessary and sufficient operational criterion might be invented for the much more abstract and far more important notion of grammaticalness. The unacceptable grammatical sentences often

> cannot be used, for reasons having to do not with grammar, but rather with memory limitations, intonational and stylistic factors, "iconic" elements of discourse.
>
> *(pp. 10–11)*

Thus, grammaticality is an abstract notion and cannot be observed or tested directly. A judgment of acceptability, on the other hand, is an act of performance, and judgment tests of the kind used in linguistics as well as second language research are subject to the same needs for experimental rigor as any other experimental task. The term *grammaticality judgment* is, therefore, misleading in that there is no test of grammaticality. What there is, instead, is a test of acceptability from which one infers grammaticality. Put differently, researchers use one (acceptability) to infer the other (grammaticality).

However, in the linguistics literature as well as the second language literature, these two terms are often used without a careful consideration of their differences. This is the case even for those who, as Myers (2009a) notes, "should know better" (p. 412). For instance, Schütze succumbs to this temptation in his classic 1996 book on this topic. "Perhaps more accurate terms for grammaticality judgments would be *grammaticality sensations* and *linguistic reactions*. Nonetheless, for the sake of familiarity I shall continue using traditional terminology, on the understanding that it must not be taken literally" (p. 52). Nearly 20 years after Schütze's important book on the topic, Schütze and Sprouse (2013) acknowledge the inappropriateness of the term *grammaticality judgment*:

> Speakers' reactions to sentences have traditionally been referred to as grammaticality judgments, but this term is misleading. Since a grammar is a mental construct not accessible to conscious awareness, speakers cannot have any impressions about the status of a sentence with respect to that grammar; rather, in Chomsky's (1965) terms, one should say their reactions concern *acceptability*, that is, the extent to which the sentence sounds "good" or "bad" to them. Acceptability judgments (as we refer to them henceforth) involve explicitly asking speakers to "judge" (i.e. report their spontaneous reaction concerning) whether a particular string of words is a possible utterance of their language, with an intended interpretation either implied or explicitly stated.
>
> *(pp. 27–28)*

Similarly, Ionin and Zyzik (2014), citing work by Cowart (1997), opt for the term *acceptability judgment task* in their review article, even though many of the studies they discuss use the term *grammaticality judgment task*.

Myers (2009a) presented data based on a survey from *Linguistics and Language Behavior Abstracts* (*LLBA*) of linguistic studies mentioning grammaticality or acceptability judgments over a period from 1973 to 2007. The search input was "syntactic judgment experiments and grammaticality" and "syntactic judgment experiments and acceptability." It is interesting to note the preponderance of the term *grammaticality judgment* particularly in the early years, although in more recent studies, there appears to be a switch to the more appropriate term *acceptability judgment*. In Figure 1.1, we present an expansion of those data to cover the period of 1972–2015. In Chapter 2, we present a comparable chart for second language research.

What do acceptability judgments reflect? Schütze and Sprouse (2013) describe acceptability judgments as perceptions of acceptability (p. 28). They point out that they are "not intrinsically less informative than, say, reaction time measures—in fact, many linguists would argue that they are more informative for the purposes of investigating the grammatical system" (p. 28). In other words, they are a useful tool for some purposes (namely understanding the grammatical system of a language), although they may be less useful for others.

We have struggled with which term to use in this book, very much wanting to use the theoretically correct term *acceptability judgment*, but also wishing to reflect reality in the use of these terms. We finally decided to use the term *acceptability judgments* throughout this book. We came to this decision in part to be theoretically consistent and in part as a way of ensuring that the field of L2 research as a whole adopts appropriate terminological usage and in so doing has a deeper understanding of the construct of *judgment data*. We also frequently resort to the phrase *judgment task* or *judgment data* to reflect a more encompassing view of types of judgment tasks.

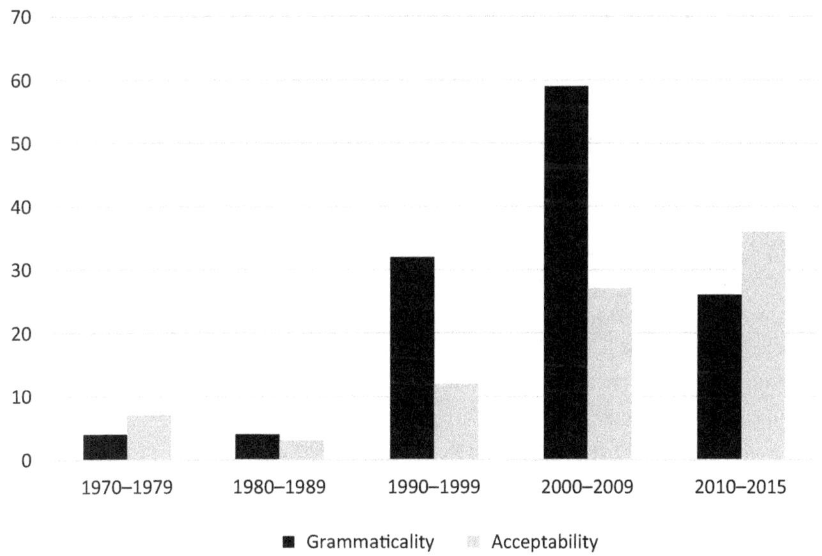

FIGURE 1.1 Syntactic judgment experiments, 1972–2015 (Linguistics)

1.2.2. Usefulness of Judgment Data

Despite the fact that opinions on acceptability judgments are often strong, and sometimes strongly negative (see Schütze, 1996; Marantz, 2005; Myers, 2009a, 2009b; Cowart, 1997), they remain a common method for data elicitation in both linguistics and second language research. Sprouse, Schütze, and Almeida (2013), in a survey of articles that appeared in *Linguistic Inquiry* from 2001–2010, estimate that data from approximately 77% of those articles came from some form of acceptability judgment task. Why are these data needed? We will deal with this topic in greater detail when we turn to discussions of second language data, but at this point we refer to early uses of judgment data.

In general, within the field of linguistics, judgment data collection has been informal. This has been the case where linguists are conducting field work in an attempt to document the grammar of an unknown language, or where they use their own intuitions about possible and impossible sentences in a language to make particular theoretical claims, or when they use the "*Hey Sally*" method, where a colleague down the hall is called upon for a judgment (Ferreira, 2005, p. 372). In linguistics, fieldwork has occupied an important place, particularly in documenting languages where there may be little written information. For example, consider the situation when a linguist is interested in understanding the grammar of a language that has no written documentation. One way of determining the grammar of that language is to transcribe all of the spoken data over a period of time; this would be not only time-consuming but also inefficient. Of course, in today's research world, corpora can give a wide range of sentences and utterances, but there are languages where corpora are not available or where they are limited. And, even where corpora are readily available, one is often left with the question of why *x* has not been heard. Is it because of happenstance, or is it because *x* is truly impossible in that language? It is in this sense that written or spoken data are insufficient; they simply do not capture the full range of grammatical sentences, and they provide insufficient information about what is outside the grammar of a language. The alternative is to probe the acceptability (or potential lack thereof) of certain possible sentences, attempting to determine whether they are or are not part of the possible sentences of that language. To do so, one typically asks native speakers of a language for their judgments about certain sentences.

Using judgment data allows linguists to "peel off" unwanted data, such as slips of the tongue that have gone uncorrected in spoken discourse, for example, when someone says *He wanted to know if she teached yesterday*. The speaker perhaps realized right away that *he wanted to know if she taught yesterday* was what he should have said, but in order to keep the flow of the conversation going, or for any number of reasons, the speaker does not make the change. If someone were doing field work on this "exotic" language, the conclusion would be that the first sentence was acceptable in English.

1.2.3. Reliability

A common informal use of judgment data has been the "ivory tower" use, where linguists provide their own examples of what is and what is not acceptable and develop theoretical positions on that basis. In an early article, Hill (1961) showed that the intuitions of Chomsky on certain sentences were not borne out by others. He recognized early on that some of Chomsky's statements (e.g., about the behavior of "any speaker of English") "constitute predictions which invite experimental verification" (p. 2). For example, Chomsky (1957) had predicted that sentences such as Example 1 would be read by native speakers with normal sentence intonation (p. 16), but sentences such as Example 2 would be read with falling intonation on each word (p. 16) (i.e., like a list).

Example 1. Colorless green ideas sleep furiously.
Example 2. Furiously sleep ideas green colorless.

Hill asked members of his academic community to read these (and other) sentences, finding that Chomsky's predictions were not borne out. From this, coupled with other data he collected, Hill concluded that isolated sentences are not a good source for informal[1] data collection (see Chomsky, 1961, for his response to this article). It is also the case that sentences thought to be unacceptable may be considered by some speakers to be somewhat acceptable; we will discuss this issue further in this chapter in Section 1.2.7.

Chomsky and Lasnik (1977, p. 491) raised the question of the reliability of linguists' judgments. In talking about arguments made by Bresnan (1977), they stated:

> We find these cases rather marginal and have little faith in our judgments. Bresnan's argument rests on the assumption that there is a crucial difference between [example *x* and *y*], but no crucial difference between [*x'* and *y'*]. We are skeptical that any persuasive argument can be based on such data, and the crucial judgments here seem to us extremely dubious if not mistaken. However, since this is the only remaining argument that has been proposed in objection to a surface filter analysis of the sort we have suggested, we will pursue it, despite the questionable character of the data.
>
> *(p. 104)*

Even though the informal collection of judgment data has been the mainstay of the field, there are some who argue that the informality undermines findings and compromises the rigor generally found in cognitive science (see Featherston, 2007; Ferreira, 2005 for discussions). Formal experimental data both support and refute informal judgment data. For example, Cowart (1997, pp. 18–19) reports on experimental data on *that*-trace effects. The issue at hand is the possibility/non-possibility of the following English sentences.

Example 3. I wonder who you think likes John.
Example 4. I wonder who you think John likes.
Example 5. I wonder who you think that likes John.
Example 6. I wonder who you think that John likes.

Theoretical conclusions have been drawn from informal judgments of these sentences. Cowart, in an empirical study (with different orderings of sentences) collected data from 32 participants. He found support for the informal judgments, although he also suggested that the subtleties stemming from experimentally elicited data are often not picked up by linguists. In particular, Sentences 3 and 4 were deemed equally acceptable, whereas Sentence 5 was more unacceptable than 6; both were less acceptable than 3 and 4 (see findings from Featherston, 2005, who had similar results from German).

On the other side of the debate is work by Featherston (2007), who argued that "insufficient attention to data can lead syntactic theory astray" (p. 277). Featherston presented data from Grewendorf (1988) on object coreference. Grewendorf (translated from German by Featherston) remarked about his confidence in his own intuitions: "The generalization can be illustrated once again in the following contrast, for someone who has a feeling for subtle, but nevertheless unequivocal grammaticality differences" (p. 273). In an earlier paper, Grewendorf (1985) also relied on his own intuitions, stating: "Even if the relevant examples are sometimes somewhat difficult to follow semantically, the syntactic intuitions of the regularities established seem to me to be relatively clear" (translated by Featherston, 2007, p. 273). Grewendorf used these intuitions to draw theoretical conclusions about anaphoric binding. Featherston tested these conclusions in an experimental format in which 26 participants gave judgments of syntactic structures using magnitude estimation[2] (Bard, Robertson, & Sorace, 1996). The results of Featherston's study did not support the "clear" intuitions of a linguist: "There is no visible effect which would support a hierarchy of binding relations" (p. 274). He goes on to say:

> The judgments of an individual are revealed to be inadequate as a basis for theory development. Finer data is required in part because of the number of effects which influence judgements in these examples (see Featherston, 2002) and because some of these effects are relatively modest, perhaps smaller than the random "noise" factor in the individual's judgements.
>
> *(p. 274)*

Another argument made by Featherston in his 2007 paper against the adequacy of linguists' own judgments is the following:

> It is also insufficient to take judgements uncritically from the literature and build upon them, since the literature is full of examples of dubious practice. I have on my desk a paper by an author with a PhD from MIT and a job at a prestigious university. The main point of the article rests upon the interpretation of two structures (both in English and German). But the author is not a native speaker of either of these languages and these critical readings are simply unavailable to me or anyone I have asked. Some related structures do show the intended readings, as do the original examples given in the first paper on the issue 25 years ago, but the author has simply not checked the facts. This is not a new problem. Greenbaum (1977) comments, "All too often the data in linguistics books and articles are dubious, which in turn casts doubt on the analyses. Since analyses usually build on the results of previous analyses, the effect of one set of dubious data left unquestioned can have far-reaching repercussions that are not easily perceived." Practice in syntax has not changed in thirty years, it would seem.
>
> *(p. 278)*[3]

1.2.4. Disconnects

In many of his writings, Labov (1975) points to the frequent disconnect between judgments (even in published works) of sentences and the way those same sentences are assessed by non-linguists. He expressed skepticism at the reliability of judgments especially in those instances when the judger and theory producer were one and the same. His was an early voice in promoting empirically based research methods alongside the use of traditional intuitional data. In addition, he noted that behaviors and judgments do not always match; in other words, those who judge a given sentence as ungrammatical may produce that same sentence. Labov (1996) reports data from interviews in which the well-known positive *anymore* phenomenon was the focus of inquiry. Essentially, this phenomenon reflects the use of *anymore* to roughly mean *nowadays* or to refer to something that is true in today's world, but perhaps was not true in the past. In Labov's interview data were instances of individuals who said that these sentences were not possible or even that they had never heard them. However, in the interview, the same individuals uttered the following:

Example 7. Do you know what's a lousy show anymore? Johnny Carson. (stated by a 58-year-old builder raised in West Philadelphia)

Example 8. Anymore, I hate to go in town anymore.

Example 9. Well, anymore, I don't think there is any proper way 'cause there's so many dialects. (both 8 and 9 were uttered by a 42-year-old Irish woman)

What these examples suggest is that, at least for naïve respondents, there is often a lack of ability to give intuitional judgments that correspond to their actual use of language.

Others (e.g., Carroll, Bever, & Pollack, 1981; Nagata, 1991) have found variability within individuals at different times and/or with different conditions. Examples such as these have been used to call into question the reliability of the methodology.

Even when informal and formal data collection results coincide, there may be subtleties that one misses with informal collection. This position is exemplified by Wasow and Arnold (2005), who conducted an empirical study (questionnaires and corpus analysis) on 1) object placement in verb particle constructions (*The children took everything we said in/The children took in everything we said/The children took all our instructions in/The children took in all our instructions*), 2) complexity (*everything we said* versus *all our instructions*), 3) dative alternation (*The company sends what Americans don't buy to subsidiaries in other countries/The company sends subsidiaries in other countries what Americans don't buy/The company sends any domestically unpopular products to subsidiaries in other countries/The company sends subsidiaries in other countries any domestically unpopular products*), and 4) heavy NP shift (*Nobody reported where the accident took place to the police/Nobody reported to the police where the accident took place/Nobody reported the location of the accident to the police/Nobody reported to the police the location of the accident*). Their data, which specifically focused on how length and complexity influence the ordering of constituents (postverbal), demonstrated how corpus data and judgment data (which they refer to as questionnaire data) can be brought to bear to understand ordering. They further argue that linguistics-based research must be subject to the same "methodological constraints typical of all scientific work" (p. 1495). Intuitional data are useful for theory construction, but data-driven approaches are also needed.

1.2.5. Rigor in Research Methods

We pointed out earlier that in many cases linguistic research has used judgment data quite informally, namely, by linguists using themselves or other linguists as models. More recently, scholars have recognized the need to treat judgment data as a method of eliciting data that is no different from other methods.

In arguing against relying on linguists' own judgments, Wasow and Arnold (2005) take the position that data reflecting intuitions have been "tacitly granted a privileged position in generative grammar" (p. 1482), by which they mean that standards common to neighboring disciplines have not been maintained by linguists (e.g., sufficient sample size, random presentation, double blinding, appropriate statistical analysis). They cite Smith (2000), who makes the strong claim that "language should be analysed by the methodology of the natural sciences, and there is no room for constraints on linguistic inquiry beyond those typical of all scientific work" (p. vii).

Ferreira (2005) further argues in favor of the need for rigorous research methods in linguistics. One of the arguments she makes relates to the Minimalist Program (MP) within generative linguistics. "The empirical foundation for the MP is almost exclusively intuition data obtained from highly trained informants (i.e., the theorists themselves)" (p. 370). She argues that while this might have been acceptable in earlier times, it is unacceptable at a time when there are many ways of understanding and eliciting linguistic data. With more "powerful methodologies" (p. 371), the use of "armchair theories" (p. 370), or even the "Hey Sally method" (p. 372), are no longer acceptable if one wants to maintain a connection between linguistic theory and cognitive science.

Marantz (2005) makes a similar comment. "Judgments of, e.g., grammaticality **are** behavioral data, and the connection between such data and linguistic theory should follow the standard scientific methodology of cognitive science" (p. 432). In Marantz's view, there is a difference between data based on (informal) judgments and those stemming from experimental work. The typical linguist, he argues, sees examples (grammatical and ungrammatical sentences) not as "data" in the typical sense that a cognitive scientist conceives of data, but rather as "standing in" for potential data. Judgments may be considered "summaries of the results of experiments the reader could perform at home" (p. 432). In that sense, informal judgments from linguists are a type of meta-data.

1.2.6. In Defense of Acceptability Judgments

As is clear from earlier discussions, acceptability judgments have been called into question despite being the mainstay of linguistic theory construction. Some researchers have suggested that they be discarded for other, more modern methods. For instance, Branigan and Pickering (2017) argue in favor of syntactic priming experiments instead of acceptability judgments to determine linguistic representation.[4] Sprouse and Almeida (2017a), while not refuting the value of priming data, rebut the challenges made by Branigan and Pickering. In particular, they discuss six claims (pp. 2–3). Below, we present four of the claims (in bold) and summarize Sprouse and Almeida's responses to them.

a. ***Linguists standardly ask a single informant about the acceptability of a few sentences.***

   Branigan and Pickering voice concerns about small sample sizes and investigator bias. However, empirical evidence presented by Sprouse et al. (2013) suggests that larger sample sizes corroborated results presented in a prominent linguistic journal at 95% level. In other words, the sample size generally used by linguists introduced little error when measured against the responses from larger sample sizes.

b. ***Acceptability judgments are highly susceptible to theoretical cognitive bias because linguists tend to use professional linguists as participants.***

Sprouse and Almeida (2017a) argue that this is not a persistent problem. They report studies that compare "naïve and expert populations" (p. 2) and conclude that "these results are not what one would expect if AJs were highly susceptible to cognitive bias" (p. 2). For example, Dabrowska (2010) found that experts often judged sentences as having greater acceptability than naïve judges even when those judgments went against their "theoretical commitments" (p. 2).

c. ***Acceptability judgments are susceptible to differences in instructions.***

As Sprouse and Almeida (2017a) point out, Cowart (1997) found that manipulation of instructions does not change the patterns of judgments. However, while this may be the case for data from native speakers of a language, the situation for second language learners may be different. In Chapter 4, we provide examples of different types of instructions for second language learners.

d. ***Acceptability judgments are impacted by sentence processing effects.***

Sprouse and Almeida acknowledge that this may be an issue. However, they point out that this is a similar problem in other experimental settings: "To the extent that AJs are impacted by sentence processing, it appears as though the effects can be dealt with like any other source of noise in an experimental setting" (p. 3). We return to this issue in the following chapter, because the same claim has been made for L2 acceptability judgments.

Importantly, Sprouse and Almeida (2017b) also provided empirical findings in defense of acceptability judgments. Their goal was to present "an empirical estimation of the sensitivity of formal acceptability judgment experiments in detecting theoretically interesting contrasts between different sentence types" (p. 31). What they are concerned with is the statistical power that is found in different kinds of experimental designs: 1) dichotomous (i.e., binary), 2) two-alternative forced-choice (essentially a preference task), 3) Likert scale (7-point), and 4) magnitude estimation. Sprouse and Almeida created a large database that included a range of participants from published studies as well as a range of effect sizes, and measured those studies against responses from 144 participants for each task. Of their results, we highlight a few here. First, the most sensitive of the four elicitation types for the detection of differences was the preference task. Likert and magnitude estimation were similar in sensitivity. The dichotomous choice task was the least sensitive. To address their main concern, they conclude that their results "suggest that acceptability judgment experiments with relatively small sample sizes are actually relatively well powered to detect many of the phenomena currently in the syntax literature" (p. 32). Note, however, that the conclusions may not be the same for second language learners. For instance, results may depend on proficiency levels because the nuanced differences that linguists deal with are in most instances beyond the abilities of many L2 learners. For more information regarding Sprouse and Almeida's work, researchers can access the following website: *www.sprouse.uconn.edu*. Available at that site is

> a database of information regarding the rate of statistical detection (our proxy measure of statistical power) that covers a substantial portion of possible experimental designs in syntax, and that is freely available to syntacticians . . . for use in the design and analysis of judgment experiments.
>
> *(Sprouse & Almeida, 2017b, p. 28)*

Sprouse and Almeida (2012) investigated the reliability of textbook data by comparing traditional judgment responses (binary) with judgments based on magnitude estimation. All participants came from Amazon Mechanical Turk. In the first data set, there were 240 naïve participants, and in the second, there were 200. The participants judged sentences (in some cases slightly modified) from a standard syntax textbook. The authors found only a slight divergence (2%) between what they refer to as traditional methods (dichotomous judgments) and formal experimental methods (magnitude estimation). Their goal was not to argue against formal experimental methods but to make the point that with such a strong convergence (98%), one should not discard traditional elicitation methods.

In this section and the preceding one, we have presented a brief synopsis of controversies about intuitional data that originate with linguists themselves. However, the use of informal data gathering, or so-called *armchair intuitions*, has never been part of the L2 data-gathering tradition. Because L2 learners do not necessarily share an L2 grammar, an informal judgment from one does not necessarily reflect judgments from others. In other words, there is not a community of speakers who can be said to have a shared grammar. When native speaker intuitions are used, they are typically included as a formal comparison group. We turn now to an issue that is more directly relevant to L2 research, namely that of the gradient nature of judgment data.

1.2.7. Gradience of Linguistic Data

Thus far we have mainly discussed binary, absolute judgments; that is, is a sentence acceptable or not? For example, a sentence such as the one in Example 10 below (from Ferreira, 2005, p. 371 who cites Akmaijian & Heny, 1975 as the original source) is without a doubt ungrammatical, and one does not need an experiment, sophisticated or otherwise, to make that determination.

Example 10. John sold the car at Bill near forty dollars.

However, it is crucial to recognize the gradient nature of judgments. For instance, consider Example 11. In the linguistic literature, sentences such as these are often marked with ? or *? to indicate that an utterance is neither totally acceptable nor totally unacceptable.

Example 11. *? *She recommended me a good book.*

Consider also sentences such as those in Examples 12–13 (cited in Ferreira, 2005, p. 371).

Example 12. Which car did John ask how Mary fixed?
Example 13. Who did John ask which car fixed?

Are both unacceptable? Is one more acceptable/unacceptable than the others? In comparing 12 and 13, both are ungrammatical, but 13 is undoubtedly worse than 12. In other words, gradience in judgments is expected.

Similarly, Levelt et al. (1977) point out that even though the main goal of linguistic-based research is to determine the set of grammatical sentences (and set them apart from the ungrammatical ones), there is the issue of *semigrammaticality* that must be dealt with. Chomsky (1965) recognized degrees of acceptability and tried to account for the continuous nature of judgments by examining the type of rule violation involved (cf. p. 150). But the explanation for gradience is not completely clear. There are at least two possible sources for gradience in judgments: either gradience is a reflection of gradience in grammars, or gradience is a reflection of the fact that judgments are a type of performance, and, as with any type of performance, gradience is to be expected.

Over the years there have been arguments on both sides: 1) grammars are continuous (and thus the source of gradience lies in the grammar), or 2) grammars are dichotomous (and thus the source of gradience lies in performance issues). For example, Bever and Carroll (1981), Gerken and Bever (1986), and Newmeyer (2007), among others, have argued that one can maintain a dichotomous view of grammar (sentences are grammatical or not) and attribute the well-established fact of gradient judgments to issues of performance. Others, such as Ross (1972) and Lakoff (1973), on the other hand, argue for the continuous nature of language ("squish," in Ross' terms) and, therefore, claim that the gradient nature of judgments is a reflection of the gradience in language. Lakoff, in particular, argues for the mental reality of "fuzzy" grammars, that is, grammars of a non-dichotomous nature. He concludes (p. 271):

a. Rules of grammar do not simply apply or fail to apply; rather they apply to a degree.
b. Grammatical elements are not simply members or nonmembers of grammatical categories; rather they are members to a degree.
c. Grammatical constructions are not simply islands or non-islands; rather they may be islands to a degree.
d. Grammatical constructions are not simply environments or non-environments for rules; rather they may be environments to a degree.
e. Grammatical phenomena form hierarchies which are largely constant from speaker to speaker, and in many cases, from language to language.
f. Different speakers (and different languages) will have different acceptability thresholds along these hierarchies.

More recently, Sorace and Keller (2005) conducted a review of studies in which gradient acceptability judgments are found and argue that the best way to account for this phenomenon is to assume gradient grammars. From a slightly different perspective, Bresnan (2007) and Bresnan and Ford (2010) suggest a probabilistic model of language (involving the likelihood a given structure is to occur in spoken or written discourse), deriving much of their research from large corpora. They examined the dative alternation, as in *Ted denied Kim the opportunity to march* versus *Ted denied the opportunity to march to Kim* (Bresnan & Ford, 2010, p. 171); these are commonly viewed as representing grammatical and ungrammatical sentences respectively. Participants were given context, as in Example 14. These were based on corpora, with one of the choices being the actual continuation and the other a constructed alternative (Bresnan & Ford, 2010, pp. 184–185):

Example 14. Context: I'm in college, and I'm only twenty-one but I had a speech class last semester, and there was a girl in my class who did a speech on home care of the elderly. And I was so surprised to hear how many people, you know, the older people, are like, fastened to their beds so they can't get out just because, you know, they wander the halls. And they get the wrong medicine, just because, you know,

a. the aides or whoever just give the wrong medicine to them.
b. the aides or whoever just give them the wrong medicine.

Judgments were made on a scale of 1–100, where the rating added up to 100. Equal values could be assigned to the two sentences (i.e., 50–50), or responses could be preferential with any combination as long as the total between the two added up to 100. Their results showed that corpus probabilities fit well with the sensitivities of native speakers. Gradience of judgments reflect probabilistic knowledge.

1.2.8. Who Are Judgments Collected From?

The selection of participants who provide judgments has been a source of some concern. The discussion has mainly centered on whether linguists and non-linguists (and, to some extent, subcategories of non-linguists) provide different judgments. This concern goes back to at least Greenbaum (1973), who, using non-linguists as participants, replicated a study by Elliot, Legum, and Thompson (1969, as cited in Greenbaum). In the Elliot et al. study, the data on syntactic variation came primarily from linguists (21 of 27 respondents). The results from non-linguists (Greenbaum's study) differed from those of the linguists in the Elliot et al. study.

In an interesting study, Spencer (1973) took published judgments (by six linguists) as his baseline. He presented the sentences from these published works to naïve participants and nonnaïve participants (graduate students in psychology, speech, or linguistics) and asked for dichotomous judgments. It is not surprising that the non-linguists' judgments differed in many instances from the judgments of linguists. Other studies have found similar differences among groups of more or less sophisticated judgments (e.g., Culbertson & Gross, 2009; Dabrowska, 2010), but see the discussion from Sprouse and Almeida (2017a) above where naïve and expert judgments did not show great differences.

1.2.9. Acceptability Judgments as Performance: Confounding Variables

As with any sort of performance measure, there can be variables that interfere with an individual's responses. A goal of much linguistic research is to determine grammatical knowledge, apart from extragrammatical issues. Sprouse (2008) refers to what he calls the "granularity problem," namely the idea that acceptability judgments cannot overcome performance effects inherent in making judgments. As he notes, "it is logically possible that the unacceptability is an epiphenomenon of human language processing" (p. 686) (see also Chomsky & Miller, 1963). Other studies (e.g., Gerken & Bever, 1986: Alexopoulou & Keller, 2007; Sprouse, Wagers, & Phillips, 2012) show similar processing limitations on judgments. Sprouse (2008), through two experimental studies, argued that the sensitivity to processing effects is not uniform, but rather, judgments on syntactic phenomena are affected differently than judgments on semantic phenomena. Cowart (1997) points to another confounding factor with regard to acceptability judgments, namely, working memory limitations, pointing out that judgments of ungrammaticality may be a result of such limitations rather than a reflection of the grammatical system.

The role of working memory vis-à-vis acceptability judgments was tested by Sprouse et al. (2012) in two experiments, one using a 7-point Likert scale of acceptability and the other magnitude estimation to collect judgment data. In addition, two working memory tests were administered. Working memory did not appear to be a confounding variable; thus, the results from their study seemingly did not provide evidence of a relationship between individuals' processing capacity and the grammatical structure under investigation. However, Hofmeister, Staum, Casasanto, and Sag (2012) provide a contrary interpretation of these results. They argue that, in fact, the constraints found in the Sprouse et al. (2012) study may actually be due to working memory capacity. Hofmeister, Jaeger, Arnon, Sag, and Snider (2013) further that argument through a paper on source ambiguity. Recognizing the inherent ambiguity involved in distinguishing between grammar and processing, they conducted a series of experiments and concluded that processing can account for at least some of their data. These factors also clearly play a role for second language learners with any investigation of complex syntax, as will become clear in subsequent chapters.

One final confound in collecting data—and this is perhaps particularly relevant to second language research—is education level. In the linguistics literature, this has received scant attention, although the studies reported above indirectly touch on this issue. In an earlier study, Mills and Hemsley (1976) collected judgments from three groups of individuals (university students, adults with three to four years of high school and adults with one to two years of high school). A participant's level of education was an important factor in making acceptability judgments. Indeed, level of education and literacy have been found to be important factors in responses to a number of commonly used measures in linguistic and psycholinguistic research (see, e.g., Juffs & Rodríguez, 2008; Reis & Castro-Caldas, 1997; Rosselli, Ardila, & Rosas, 1990).

1.3. Conclusion

This chapter has served to introduce the reader to some of the historical background of judgments as well as some of the current controversies within the field of linguistics, where the methodology originated. In the next chapter, we turn to the use of acceptability judgments in second language research.

Notes

1. The distinction between informal and formal judgment data as a dichotomy is in actuality a false distinction. Some have equated formal judgment data as coming from an experimental context, with informal data coming from asking oneself or friends, colleagues, etc. In other words, the latter is often seen as observational (including corpus data) rather than being obtained through experimental manipulation. Myers (2009b) expresses this succinctly: "informal judgment collection is itself a form of experimentation" (p. 426) and therefore "informal methods and full-fledged experimentation lie on a continuum, rather than representing radically different types of data sources" (p. 426). He acknowledges the controversy in the literature between those who argue for formal experimentation and those who, more practically, argue that one cannot engage in such experimentation for all structures of all languages. Myers' middle ground is that "formal

experimentation should be reserved only for particularly subtle patterns that informal methods cannot resolve" (p. 426).

2. Magnitude estimation will be discussed further in Chapter 4. For now, the important point is that it is a way of obtaining a more fine-grained judgment than can be obtained through binary or dichotomous judgments (i.e., is a sentence grammatical or not?). In a magnitude estimation study, participants begin with a measurement of acceptability of a sentence of their own choosing and then measure the acceptability of each subsequent sentence against the previous one.
3. Fortunately, the issue of individual judgments versus robustly designed data elicitation does not generally come up for L2 researchers given the peculiar nature of L2 judgments. However, the issue is particularly relevant in those cases where L1 judgments are being used as a type of control against which L2 judgments are being compared.
4. What is notable about this article is that the authors appear to set priming experiments in opposition to acceptability judgments. In our view, it seems unnecessary to diminish the validity of a particular experimental method in order to demonstrate the value of another.

2

JUDGMENT DATA IN L2 RESEARCH

Historical and Theoretical Perspectives

2.1. Introduction

The preceding chapter discussed the history and current controversies relevant to the use of judgments in linguistic research. The discussion should leave no doubt as to the crucial and central role that judgments about linguistic well-formedness have had and continue to have in the study of linguistics. As Sprouse (2013) notes, "acceptability judgments form a substantial portion of the empirical foundation of nearly every area of linguistics . . . and nearly every type of linguistic theory" (p. 1). The use of judgment data in second language research is similarly rich in both use and controversy. As with any methodology, their use cannot be taken for granted, and decisions about when, why, and how to use the data must be made purposefully. The goal of this chapter is to explore the theoretical issues (both historical and current) prevalent in the L2 literature.

2.2. Judgment Data in Second Language Research

2.2.1. Terminology: Grammaticality Versus Acceptability Judgments

Issues of terminology are relevant to a discussion of the use of judgment data with L2 learners in the same way as they were to a discussion of data from native speakers (NS). In Chapter 1, we presented a lengthy discussion of terminology used to describe judgment data. We also saw that in the linguistic literature, the current trend is to use the theoretically correct term *acceptability judgment* as opposed to *grammaticality judgment*, although both are still used. Figures 2.1 and 2.2 parallel the findings in Chapter 1 (Figure 1.1) in which historical data were presented from the field of linguistics. The first of these (Figure 2.1) took the same search criteria from LLBA presented in Figure 1.1. Figure 2.2 includes a more extended database (approximately 300 studies and approximately 380 actual experiments using judgment data) that comes from research by Plonsky, Marsden, Crowther, Gass, and Spinner (in press). The data included in these studies come from empirical studies published in peer-reviewed journals, all listed in the Thomson Reuters Citation Index.[1]

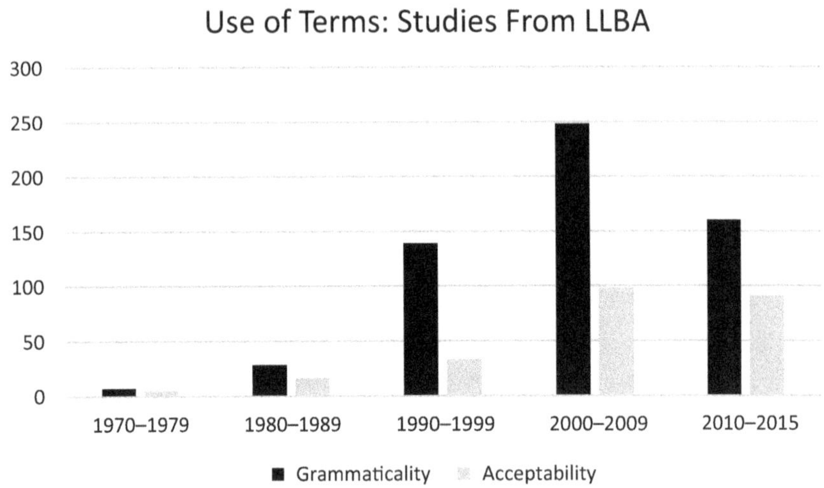

FIGURE 2.1 Syntactic judgment experiments in second language research from 1972–2015

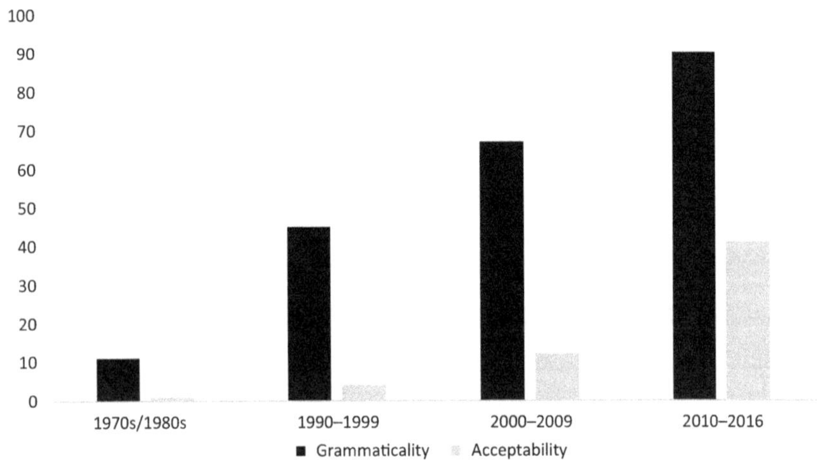

FIGURE 2.2 Terms used based on Plonsky et al. database

In both graphs, it is clear that unlike in the field of linguistics, where the term *acceptability judgment* is becoming more common, there is still a preponderance of use of the term *grammaticality judgment* in L2 research, although the ratio has changed over the past 40–50 years. Considering Figure 2.2, one can see that in the first decades (1970s, 1980s, and 1990s), in 92% of the studies *grammaticality judgment* is the preferred term; in the first decade of the current century, 85% of studies used *grammaticality judgment*; and, in the past few years, that percentage has dipped to 69%. Interestingly, in most instances, authors use one or the other without a justification; as a result, there appears to be random use of one term over the other. An early acknowledgement of this difference comes from the article by Schachter, Tyson, and Diffley (1976), in which the authors discuss the theoretical difference, but then state "we used the phrase *grammaticality judgment* to mean a judgment elicited from a learner. Our loose use of this term will perhaps be forgiven since no argument depends on it" (p. 71). Similarly, Birdsong (1992) made it clear in a footnote that *grammaticality* and *acceptability* are not synonymous:

> It is widely recognized that grammaticality and acceptability are not synonymous, and that there are serious problems with eliciting judgments and using them as evidence for grammatical competence.
>
> *(p. 714)*

Throughout his article, however, both are used (*acceptability* more than *grammaticality*). More recently, Ionin and Zyzik, 2014 wrote, referring back to Cowart (1997), "experimental tasks can test the acceptability of a given sentence by speakers, and the speakers' judgments can consequently be used to make inferences about grammaticality" (p. 38). They also point out, however, that the terms *grammaticality judgment* and *acceptability judgment* "are often used interchangeably in the literature to mean a task in which participants are presented with one sentence at a time and asked to judge its grammaticality" (p. 38). Thus, we see variation in the L2 literature in the same way as in the linguistic literature.

2.2.2. L2 Versus L1 Knowledge

Judgment data typically serve two very different purposes. First, they can be used to investigate theoretical principles of Language. That is, they can be used to understand what is and what is not within the confines of a particular language, or more generally, to understand the nature of possible human languages. This is typical of the linguistic literature described in Chapter 1. The second purpose is to understand acquisition by considering developmental paths and by determining what language learners take to be possible grammars. This is the case in both L1 and L2 acquisition research, although judgment data are used less frequently in L1 acquisition research, partially because of challenges of using them with young children. Second language judgment data are fairly commonly used for understanding the development of interlanguage (IL).

Judgment data from fully developed speakers of a native language and judgment data from language learners are different in several ways. First, with research on fully developed speakers of a native language, the responses are more likely to be homogeneous, because one can assume a community of speakers with similar grammars. That is, the researcher is collecting data about a specific language. With child language acquisition, there may be more variation in responses because each child is still in the process of creating his or her own grammar; however, the starting and finishing points for each speaker are similar. On the other hand, with second language learners, the linguistic starting and finishing points may vary widely. Learners may have different first languages, different exposure to input and types of instruction, and different levels of proficiency at the time of data collection. Unless learners are at very high levels of proficiency, their ILs are still likely to be in flux. Thus, a greater deal of heterogeneity is to be expected.

The second area of difference has to do with what is being asked. Asking second language learners about the well-formedness of a sentence in the language they are learning is not at all the same as asking someone about the well-formedness of a sentence in his/her native language. When collecting information about what is possible in someone's native language, researchers ask for judgments about that language, and inferences are then made about the grammaticality of a linguistic form in that language; what is being tapped is a system over which speakers have automatized control. Importantly, inferences are made about the same system that is being asked about. However, with speakers and learners of a second language, the picture is different; judgments are asked about the language being learned (the target language [TL]) with inferences being made about a developing system, namely one's interlanguage. To give an example, if a researcher is conducting research on L2 relative clauses, learners might be asked to judge the sentence *That's the man I saw yesterday*. If learners judge that sentence to be incorrect and change it to *That's the man I saw him yesterday*, we are likely to conclude that that speaker's IL obligatorily has resumptive pronouns. We have therefore asked a question about the target language—in this case, English—and have made an inference about a different linguistic system (an IL). We schematize this difference in Figures 2.3 and 2.4.

As is apparent from Figures 2.3 and 2.4, judgment data reflect very different phenomena in adult native language and second language research, although these differences are not always acknowledged when judgment data are used.[2]

One could consider other configurations in L2 research designs. For example, in an investigation of the role of the L1, a researcher could include sentences that target features in both the TL and the native language (NL), with inferences then being made about the IL. This is schematized in Figure 2.5.

Thus, it must be acknowledged at the outset that the use of judgment data in second language research presents unique concerns. The judgments of an L2 learner are different in fundamental ways from those of adult native speakers of

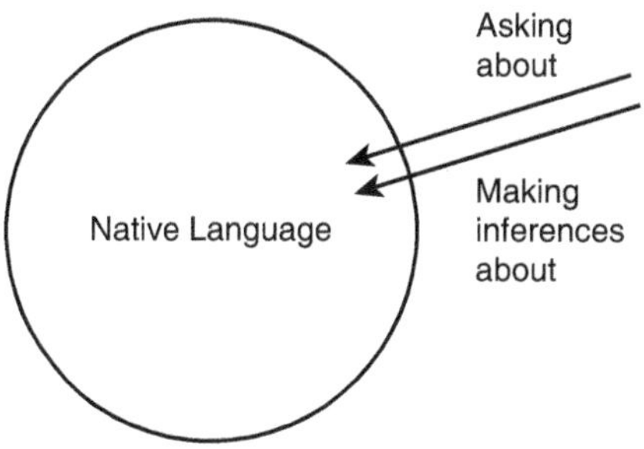

FIGURE 2.3 Adult native language judgments

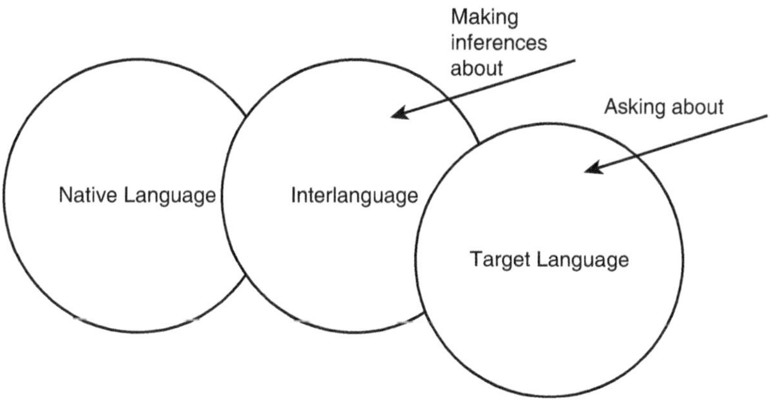

FIGURE 2.4 L2 judgments

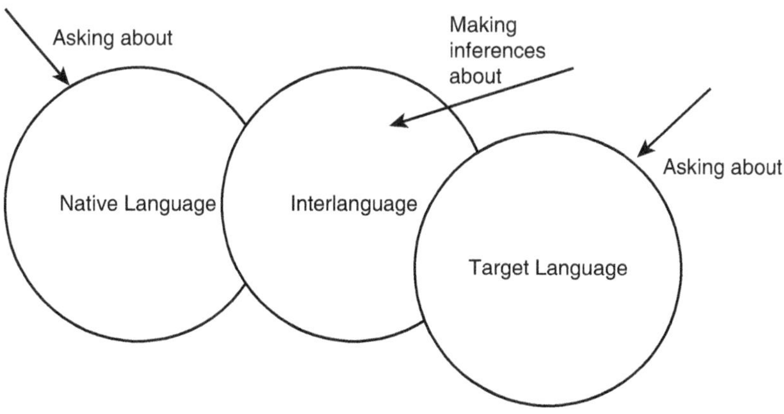

FIGURE 2.5 Schematic view when incorporating both NL and TL in design

a language. The situation is exacerbated at the stage of data analysis, which we discuss in Chapter 6.

Briefly, in L2 research, experiments are typically developed with two types of sentences in mind: grammatical and ungrammatical. However, in so doing, researchers are looking at the data from the researcher's perspective or, more aptly put, from the perspective of the TL, when in reality the goal is to understand what a learner knows of the TL. We return to this issue in Section 2.3.3 in reference to the comparative fallacy (Bley-Vroman, 1983).

2.3. L2 Judgment Data: A Brief History

Second language research has often adopted and adapted research methodologies from other disciplines. Judgments are no exception and have been used since the early days of L2 research. This is particularly the case given the overwhelmingly linguistic focus of second language research in at least the early days of L2 research. For years, the role of intuitional judgments was a subject of controversy, and the literature was replete with studies using what were most often referred to as grammaticality judgments. The use was often accompanied by a justification for their use.[3]

2.3.1. The Value of Judgment Data

Along with the use of judgment data comes debate, with a few researchers arguing that judgment data should be avoided entirely. Selinker (1972) was an early scholar to question the usefulness of judgments for the field of SLA. In his 1972 paper, he made this clear when he said that scholars should "focus our analytical attention upon *the only observable data to which we can relate theoretical predictions:* the utterances which are produced when the learner attempts to say sentences of a target language" (pp. 213–214). Selinker elaborated his belief, saying "the only observable data from meaningful performance situations we can establish as relevant . . . are . . . IL utterances produced by the learner" (p. 214). With these statements, he effectively ruled out the appropriateness of judgment data. He explicitly claimed that judgment data were inappropriate for second language research, because researchers "will gain information about another system, the one the learner is struggling with, i.e., the TL" (p. 213) (see Gass & Polio, 2014, for further discussion of this issue). This is precisely the problem addressed in relation to the discussion of Figure 2.4.

Corder (1973) took a different perspective and argued that if we truly wanted an understanding of what it means to know a second language, intuitional data had to be included. Similar to what we outlined in Figures 2.3 and 2.4, in his view learners were native speakers of their own language, their interlanguage. From this perspective, each learner has an error-free system, and it is that system that researchers are attempting to get data about. As he noted, a learner has "intuitions about the grammaticality of his language which are potentially investigable" (p. 36).

Corder's work was particularly important, in that he did not advocate only for intuitional or judgment data. Rather, he recognized that one had to use multiple sources of data. Those sources included what Selinker (1972) referred to as *observable data* or data from *meaningful performance situations*, as noted above, as well as other data sources, such as data from judgments. Corder assigns a different role to each. Data stemming from learner production serves the purpose of hypothesis creation. But this does not suffice when trying to put together a picture of L2 linguistic knowledge. Intuitional data come into play when researchers need to validate those hypotheses. In other words, the two data sources (performance and intuitions), in Corder's view, need to be considered together, so that researchers' descriptions of interlanguages match the intuitions of learners. In Corder's words, "to suggest otherwise is to suggest that a learner might say 'That is the form a native speaker would use, but I use this form instead'" (p. 41).

Following Selinker's influential paper, arguments appeared defending and advocating for the use of judgment data. For example, Schachter et al. (1976) emphasized the need to characterize "the learner's interlanguage, at different stages, in the acquisition of the target language" (p. 67). They further argued "we are interested in characterizing learner *knowledge* of his language, not simply learner production" (p. 67). They point out that "*no* attempt at the characterization of the learner's interlanguage which is based on collecting and organizing the utterances produced by the learner will be descriptively adequate" (p. 67). In arguing against Selinker's position, they provided the following hypothetical case:[4]

> Suppose some linguist was an adult learner of Hebrew, and that linguist was interested in characterizing his own interlanguage. It surely would be legitimate for him to consult his own intuitions (use introspective evidence) in his attempt to characterize his own interlanguage. And just as it would be legitimate for him to use his own intuitive judgments as data, so also would it be legitimate for him to use the intuitive judgments that he could elicit from other adult speakers of their interlanguages, as long as he used appropriate caution in interpreting the data.
>
> *(pp. 68–69)*

Schachter et al. considered both Corder's and Selinker's arguments, arguing that both were correct, but that both missed an important point:

> The native speaker is assumed to know the language the sentences of which he is being asked to judge. The learner is assumed to know his interlanguage, but questions have to be put to him in the target language . . . even if he does have intuitions about his interlanguage there will be sentences of the target language about which he has no intuitions.
>
> *(p. 69)*

This reflects the distinction we made earlier and schematized in Figure 2.4.

2.3.2. Indeterminacy

Schachter et al. (1976) were concerned with an additional point, what they called *indeterminacy*. Their schematization (Figure 2.6, where G = grammatical sentences and U = ungrammatical sentences) emphasized this distinction. Indeterminate knowledge is in some sense akin to those sentences typically characterized by linguists with ? or *?, suggesting that a respondent is not sure if the sentence in question is acceptable or not.

Schachter et al. conducted a study investigating relative clauses. The native languages of their participants were Arabic, Chinese, Japanese, Persian, and Spanish. To the extent possible, sentences were created based on prior production data of English from these language groups (see discussion of Figure 2.5). Specific sentences selected reflected 'malformations' produced by a specific group and not by other groups. One hundred participants responded orally to each sentence (20 participants from each of the five languages), indicating whether sentences were grammatical or not. Sentences that were outside of their sphere, namely, those that did not reflect their own production malformations, were responded to randomly, while those sentences that did reflect their production received a more consistent set of 'grammatical' responses.

2.3.3. The Comparative Fallacy

In an influential paper, Bley-Vroman (1983) discussed the *comparative fallacy*, which refers to instances in which the target grammar is the measure used to determine an interlanguage grammar. In other words, constructs are defined in terms of the target language, when in reality, the goal is to understand an interlanguage grammar. As Bley-Vroman states, the comparative fallacy is "the mistake of studying the systematic character of one language by comparing it to another" (p. 6). If one

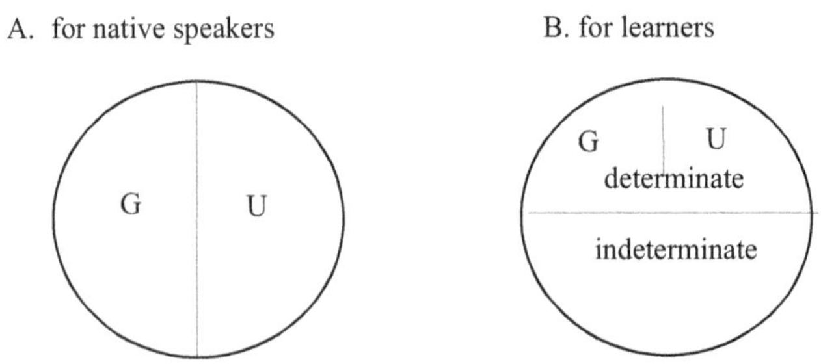

FIGURE 2.6 Set of strings of English words

Source: From "Learner intuitions of grammaticality" by J. Schachter, A. Tyson, & F. Diffley, 1976, *Language Learning, 26*, pp. 67–76. Published by Research Club in Language Learning. Reprinted by permission.

is to adhere to the notion that an interlanguage is a coherent system *où tout se tient*,[5] then one must examine and understand that system without reference to an external system. Bley-Vroman notes the following two types of studies that may reflect the comparative fallacy: 1) "any study which classifies interlanguage . . . data according to a target language scheme or depends on the notion of obligatory context or binary choice" (p. 15), or 2) "any study which uses a target language scheme to preselect data for investigation (such as a study which begins with a corpus of errors)" (p. 15). These and other studies are "likely to obscure the phenomenon under investigation" (p. 15) and "will fail to illuminate the structure of the IL" (p. 15).

Considering the role of acceptability judgments, Bley-Vroman (1990) acknowledges the fundamentally different nature of second language grammars when he suggests that

> a third class of grammaticality judgments—"indeterminate"—is needed in the description of learner language (cf. Schachter et al., 1976). This suggests that the knowledge which underlies non-native speaker performance may be incomplete (in the technical sense) and thus may be a different sort of formal object from the systems thought to underlie native speaker performance.
>
> *(p. 10)*

2.3.4. Use as Sole Measure or One of Many

Hyltenstam (1977) and Gass (1979) each used multiple sources of data, one of which was judgment data, although their rationale for using other data sources differed. In the case of Hyltenstam, the need to have a large enough database to capture "maximal variation" (p. 385) was paramount, and it was clear that production data were limited in precisely this way. He went about dealing with this problem in much the same way Corder (1973) did, by collecting production data along with judgment data. The goal of the former was to generate information about so-called problematic areas of language, and then from these data to generate hypotheses that could be verified or refuted on the basis of experimentally elicited data. This process in turn allows further hypothesis testing through additional production data. In other words, there is a cycle of production to experiment and back to production as a way of gathering detailed information about L2 learning. Sequential data sources build on one another.

Gass (1979), in her study of the L2 acquisition of relative clauses, took a different approach and collected judgment data alongside other data sources (in this case, sentence combining and written data production). She used judgment data as a primary data source due to the linguistic tradition on which her work was based, and used production data from a forced-elicitation task and a written composition task as corroborating evidence.

2.3.5. Judgment Data and Empirical Research

It was not until the early 1970s that the field of SLA began to see a large number of empirical studies, but despite this increasing interest in L2 research, judgment data were still not prevalent. Gass and Polio (2014) conducted a comparison of articles that appeared in *Language Learning*[6] and found that in the five-year period between 1967 and 1972, 11 empirical articles appeared, whereas 46 appeared in the seven years from 1973 to 1979.[7,8] However, out of these 57 empirical articles (1967–1979), only four used judgment data. Indeed, Schachter et al. (1976) had already pointed out that very few L2 studies actually used intuitional data (with Zydatiß, 1972; Ritchie, 1974 being exceptions). This is somewhat surprising given the decidedly linguistic bias in early years of L2 research. Gass (1983) argues that

> if we assume similarity to natural language, we would further suppose that they [learner languages] could be investigated through the same methods as other types of natural languages for which a chief methodological device is the use of intuitions of native speakers.
>
> *(p. 273)*

Part of the reason for the reluctance of some researchers to use judgment data is that they are, perhaps mistakenly, associated with what Sprouse (2013) refers to as "traditional" judgment collection methods, in which a researcher relies on her own intuitions or the intuitions of a few colleagues (see Marantz, 2005) rather than collecting empirical data in a rigorous fashion, as most SLA researchers attempt to do today.

Gass (1983) presents a number of other reasons why judgments were not used frequently in early L2 research. First was the close reliance on child language research and child second language acquisition research as a model, where there was an emphasis on production data. The second reason provided is discussed above and has to do with the difficulties in interpretation of judgment data from learners who are being asked to make judgments about one language, the target language, with generalizations being made about another language, the interlanguage. Finally, with fully developed adult native speakers there is generally a correspondence between production and intuitions (but see discussion in Chapter 1 for limitations on this position), while with L2 learners there may be less congruence between production and intuitions (see Spinner, 2013). An additional issue is that with learners—at least those for whom learning has taken place in a classroom context—it is more likely that metalinguistic information comes into play. Hence, true intuitional information may not be reflected in judgments. (We return to this issue in Section 2.4.2 on implicit/explicit knowledge.)

As can be seen in Figure 2.7 (modified from Plonsky et al., in press), despite the arguments for and against judgment data, the number of studies using judgments in L2 research has steadily increased over the decades since the early 1970s.

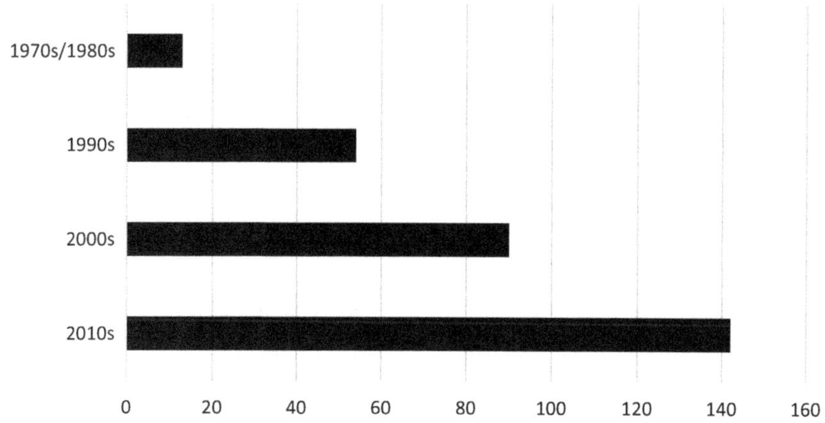

FIGURE 2.7 Use of judgments in peer-reviewed journal articles over time

Chaudron, in his 1983 review of metalinguistic judgments (using a broader criterion for inclusion in the database than the one used by Gass & Polio, 2014), reported on 22 studies between the years of 1976 and 1982 that used judgment data. Even though the selection criteria differed, it is possible to compare the two databases and conclude that, beginning in the late 1970s, there appears to be an increase in the use of this research tool. Chaudron categorized these studies by age of participants, language (L1 and L2) of participants, education of participants, the kind of task, whether the sentences were delivered aurally or visually (nearly all were visual), whether there was a time limit, whether there was training, the number of sentences included, the terminology used (grammaticality/acceptability), the scale used (dichotomous versus continuous), the feature tested, and whether there was correction required. He expressed concern about the range of "elicitation procedures and measures used" (p. 367), referring to different tasks used as well as the different measurements of those tasks. He further noted that the purpose of the studies "was to explore comparisons between subjects' judgments of, say, 'grammaticality' and 'acceptability' or 'meaningfulness,' 'ordinariness,' 'appropriateness,' 'correctness'" (p. 367). This variation still exists in the most recent survey conducted by Plonsky et al. (in press). Chaudron suggests that

> it is incumbent on the researcher to be as explicit as possible in describing the task to the subjects, and preferably to elicit reactions afterwards as to their perceived criteria for judgments . . . Such procedures, along with careful control of the test stimuli, should improve the interpretability of the results.
>
> *(p. 368)*

In his conclusion, Chaudron makes a number of important points, three of which we mention here. First, he notes that "there is reasonably clear evidence that as learners develop toward target language proficiency, their ability to match the experimenter's 'objective' norms improves" (p. 370). This suggests that judgment data indeed appropriately reflect L2 knowledge, in that, as would be predicted, they more closely approximate native speaker intuitional data as proficiency increases.

The second issue is the fact that many of the reviewed studies used other elicitation measures to validate the findings of judgment data. For instance, Schmidt and McCreary (1977) examined data from high school English teachers in Egypt and found consistency between the participants' responses on a judgment task and their production data (an issue discussed in the previous chapter, where one of the criticisms of judgment data was the lack of consistency between judgment and production data). A third positive sign is work by Gass (1994), who asked participants to judge sentences twice, with the second set of judgments occurring one week after the first. By and large, there was consistency between the two sessions. However, this finding was not uniform. For example, one student had a large discrepancy between judgments of the same sentence at the two times of data collection. In an interview following the second administration, in which the researcher attempted to probe the source of this discrepancy, the student responded, as in Example 1 (from Gass, 1994, pp. 318–319):

Example 1. R = researcher; S = student

R: Do you know why you're not so sure here?
S: I think it's definitely correct.
R: OK. Um
S: I think that happens because I have three tests tomorrow and the next day so. . .
R: So you have a lot on your mind.
S: Yeah.
R: Yeah.
S: So I'm so tired
R: That it's hard to concentrate. . .
S: Yeah.

Similarly, Kellerman (1985), referring to his own work, notes that learners base their judgments on a variety of factors and encourages researchers to "take care to control for this variation as much as possible" (p. 99). Other evidence for inconsistency comes from Liceras (1983) (reported in Ellis, 1991), who in work with early L2 learners of Spanish found differences between judgments, on the one hand, and translation and fill-in-the-blank tasks, on the other. The findings for advanced learners, however, did not follow those for beginning learners, in that production/judgment data were not as divergent. Ellis and Rathbone (1987, reported in Ellis, 1991) also found a lack of convergence between beginning L2 German judgments and production data, further supporting the claim of divergence in beginning learners and perhaps more convergence when advanced learners are the focus of inquiry.

Another important factor in the controversy regarding judgment data centers on the type of information that judgment data can provide, and whether this information is representative of a second language learner's interlanguage system. We elaborate on this issue in Section 2.4 below.

2.4. What Knowledge is Being Measured?

In this section, we highlight two common uses for judgment data: 1) understanding what is known of a second language and 2) distinguishing between implicit and explicit knowledge.

2.4.1. Measuring Knowledge of Form

The most common use for judgment data is measuring knowledge of form. Researchers have used judgment data to understand what learners know and do not know of a second/foreign language. This approach is often taken within a generativist framework by researchers who are attempting to understand the extent to which an interlanguage grammar is constrained in the same way as a natural language grammar. A review of this literature is beyond the scope of this book, but suffice it to say that judgment data are frequently used when looking at syntax and/or morphosyntax. We elaborate on this topic in Chapter 4, but the main point is that it is impossible to know what is ungrammatical for a learner through production data alone. To take what can be considered a trivial example, Italian has sentences both with and without pronouns. ("She sees" can be realized as *vede* [literally, "sees"] or *lei vede* [literally, "she sees"]). If an Italian learner of English says "she sees" in English, it is clear that she knows that pronouns *can* be used in English, but does she understand that pronouns are obligatory? Perhaps the learner operates under the assumption that pronouns are optional, but she has coincidentally only heard sentences including pronouns. Clearly, additional probing is necessary, and that is where judgment tasks (as well as other elicitation measures) can come into the picture.

A second way judgment data have been used is to test learning following an intervention (classroom or otherwise). In such instances, there is likely to be a pretest and a posttest (or even delayed posttests) to determine any knowledge changes that may have taken place as a result of the treatment.

Similar to the L1 research discussed in Chapter 1, L2 studies have compared results from different elicitation tasks, although there are few studies that compare elicitation methods for the sake of understanding which methodology more closely reflects L2 knowledge. For example, Hwang and Lardiere (2013) used an acceptability task, a preference task, and a truth-value judgment task (as well as two others) to better understand intrinsic and extrinsic plural marking by L1 English speakers with Korean as an L2. Other studies (e.g., Kupisch, 2012; Indrarathne & Kormos, 2017) also use multiple measures to determine the extent of learners' knowledge.

2.4.2. Implicit and Explicit Knowledge

The constructs of implicit and explicit knowledge have figured prominently in the L2 literature. Judgments have been used to differentiate between these two types of knowledge, with timing of responses being the major differentiating factor (see Chapter 4).[9] In current research, however, the issue of the type of knowledge that is tapped by judgment data is quite controversial.

Bialystok (1979), building on her 1978 work, claims that "the proficient use of a language, either native or non-native, depends on a complex interplay of information that is either explicitly consulted or intuitively based" (p. 81). She defines these two as follows:

> Explicit Linguistic Knowledge contains all the conscious facts the learner has about the language and the criterion of admission to this category is the ability to articulate those facts. . . . Implicit Linguistic Knowledge is the intuitive information upon which the language learner operates in order to produce responses (comprehension or production) in the target language.
>
> *(Bialystok, 1978, p. 72)*

Bialystok (1979) refers back to Vygotsky (1967), who distinguishes between "deliberate and automatic forms" (Bialystok, p. 82) on the basis of whether the language is the speaker's first or second language. For Vygotsky, native language knowledge is implicit and foreign/second language knowledge is explicit. On the other hand, for Bialystok and in current research, both types of knowledge can exist in both language knowledge contexts. What is important is that the distinction is in terms of "function rather than content" (Bialystok, 1978, p. 73). She further notes that

> a larger Implicit Linguistic Knowledge source is associated with an ability for greater fluency; a larger Explicit Linguistic Knowledge source is associated with extensive knowledge of formal aspects of the language but does not necessarily imply an ability to use this information effectively.
>
> *(p. 73)*

That is, any information can be represented in either source. It is how those sources are used for spontaneous production/comprehension that differs.

Similarly, Krashen (1982) distinguished between two constructs, *acquisition* and *learning*. *Acquisition* referred to the building of implicit knowledge, while *learning* referred to the building of explicit (and less useful) knowledge. Krashen's overall incorporation of the distinction into a complete model of second language learning suffered from a lack of clarity, but the distinction is still relevant, as is clear based on the numerous studies based on this bifurcation of knowledge types.

Bialystok was one of the early researchers to use judgment data to distinguish between these two knowledge types. In her 1979 paper, she collected data from English-speaking learners of French. She used two judgment tasks, one that forced a quick response (3 seconds per judgment) and one that allowed more time (15 seconds per judgment). Based on the results, she proposed a processing model that suggested that implicit knowledge initially drives the determination of the acceptability of a sentence, and explicit knowledge is used to further analyze those sentences that participants believe are incorrect, particularly if an additional task such as correction is included. She pointed out that her results needed to be validated against tasks that unquestionably require explicit knowledge (e.g., discrete-point achievement test) and those that unquestionably require implicit knowledge (e.g., natural conversation with native speakers) (cf. Ellis, 2005 as an example of this sort of validation).

Gass (1983) drew on Bialystok's work to interpret results from a study on intuitions. In Gass' study, judgments were collected from 21 learners of English (13 intermediate, 8 advanced). Within 24 hours following a written essay, each student's sentences (grammatical and ungrammatical in English) were extracted and presented to that student. The task was to judge each sentence as either a "good English sentence" or a "bad English sentence" followed by a correction of an error if the sentence was judged "bad." Gass speculated that

> the initial stages [of learning] represent the development of a generalized feeling of what is right or wrong. This continues to be refined so that more accurate assessments can be made. In other words, we note a gradual change from implicit to explicit knowledge where explicit knowledge reflects a learner's ability to view the language as an abstract entity.
>
> *(p. 286)*

Ellis (2009a) outlines criteria for distinguishing between the two knowledge types, three of which are mentioned below (pp. 10–15):

1. Implicit knowledge is tacit and intuitive whereas explicit knowledge is conscious.
2. Implicit knowledge is procedural whereas explicit knowledge is declarative.
3. Implicit knowledge is available through automatic processing whereas explicit knowledge is generally accessible only through controlled processing.

Ellis (2009b) operationalizes these constructs as follows: "explicit knowledge is conceptualized as involving primarily 'analyzed knowledge' (i.e., structured knowledge of which learners are consciously aware). . . . Implicit knowledge is characterized as subsymbolic, procedural and unconscious" (p. 38). He discusses seven "criterial features" (p. 38) on which these definitions rely.

1. Degree of awareness (extent to which learners are aware of their knowledge);
2. Time available (planned responses or not);
3. Focus of attention (does the task prioritize fluency or accuracy?);
4. Systematicity (the extent to which learners are consistent in their responses);
5. Certainty (how confident are learners in their responses);
6. Metalanguage (knowledge of metalinguistic terms);
7. Learnability (age of initial learning).

In an effort to determine which tasks measure implicit versus explicit knowledge, Han and Ellis (1998) conducted a study using four different elicitation measures to elicit verb complements: 1) an oral production test, 2) a timed judgment test, 3) an untimed judgment test, and 4) an interview in which participants were asked to judge sentences and then state a rule to explain the underlying grammar point. Based on a factor analysis, they found that the first two loaded on one factor and the second two on another. The factor for the first two tasks was labeled implicit knowledge and the factor for the second two tasks was labeled explicit knowledge.

Two features of judgment tasks generally figure into the controversy surrounding whether they measure implicit or explicit knowledge. The first, as noted earlier, is time pressure. In a review of judgment tasks, Loewen (2009) pointed out that allowing limited time to respond is likely to produce results that are more reflective of implicit knowledge. However, Loewen points to difficulties with creating time pressure. For example, how much time should be given, and how is that determined? There needs to be sufficient time to process the sentence, but not too much time to allow participants to access explicit knowledge. He pointed to work by Ellis (2004), who brings in issues of sentence complexity in relation to how much time is needed (e.g., more complex sentences require more time for judgments). Additionally, Purpura (2004) brings into the picture the role of test-taking anxiety, which could be generated by pressuring participants to provide responses quickly. Anxiety would therefore be another, presumably unwanted, variable.

In a partial replication of Ellis (2005), Godfroid et al. (2015) investigated NNS' (*N* = 40) and NS' (*N* = 20) processing of timed and untimed acceptability judgments in English, simultaneously tracking participants' eye-movements. Both the timed and untimed acceptability judgment tasks consisted of 68 sentences (half grammatical, half ungrammatical) composed of 17 different target linguistic structures. Participants judged each sentence as grammatical or ungrammatical and were asked to provide source attributions (e.g., intuition, rule) and confidence ratings.

Multinomial logistic regression was conducted to investigate the link between eye gaze behavior and performance on judgment items, with L1 (NS, NNS), grammaticality (Grammatical, Ungrammatical), and timing (Timed, Untimed) as predictor variables of judgments. Whereas native speakers' eye patterns remained roughly stable across timed and untimed items, non-native speakers read timed and untimed items differently; specifically, on untimed items they tended to read through sentences fully before regressing to an earlier region far more often. In addition, grammatical items featured more full read-throughs than ungrammatical items on the untimed acceptability judgment task for both NSs and NNSs. Based on their findings, the authors argue, in support of Ellis (2005), that timed and untimed acceptability judgment tasks may measure different constructs, which may be seen as implicit and explicit knowledge respectively.

The second issue discussed in Loewen (2009) is the stimulus type, that is, whether the sentences are grammatical or ungrammatical in the target language. Hedgcock (1993), in his review article, suggests different processes in judging grammatical versus ungrammatical sentences: "While some subjects may develop an impressive level of metalinguistic awareness, this sensitivity frequently appears to be asymmetrical in that a subject's demonstrated ability to detect ungrammaticalities may not match her ability to confirm grammatical L2 forms" (p. 17). However, it is more likely that the process is the same, namely that of matching a test sentence to something represented in a learner's IL grammar. What differs is the time taken to come to a determination of a match and the outcome of the matching process. A match can happen relatively quickly in the case of a sentence that is grammatical for a learner. However, if there is no immediate match, as in the case of a sentence that is not part of a learner's IL grammar, searching for a match continues (see also Bialystok, 1979) until the learner determines that a match is unlikely to be found. This process inevitably takes longer.

Ellis (2009b) reports on what is called "The Marsden Project," which expanded upon the Han and Ellis (1998) study. The study involved 17 English grammatical structures known to be problematic for L2 learners. One hundred and eleven participants completed five tasks, including a timed and an untimed judgment test. Among the results, two findings are most relevant for an understanding of the role of judgment data. First, participants appeared to respond differently to grammatical and ungrammatical sentences in the untimed judgment condition. In particular, ungrammatical sentences had a stronger correlation with the metalinguistic knowledge test, and grammatical sentences demonstrated a stronger correlation with the elicited oral imitation task. Second, confirmatory factor analysis showed that results from the oral imitation test, the oral narrative test, and the timed judgment test loaded onto one factor, and the ungrammatical sentences in the untimed condition loaded on a separate factor together with the metalinguistic knowledge test. This result suggests that the judging of ungrammatical sentences taps into more explicit knowledge, while the judging of grammatical sentences taps into more implicit knowledge (cf. Bialystok, 1979; Erlam & Loewen, 2010, for further discussion of this point).

Gutiérrez (2013) builds on Loewen's work (2009) and investigates the construct validity of judgment tasks, taking into account time pressure and stimulus type. In a study of 49 L2 Spanish learners, he collected data from two judgment tasks (timed and untimed) and a metalinguistic knowledge task. Using both principal components factor analysis and exploratory factor analysis (as well as other statistical measures), Gutiérrez concludes that grammatical and ungrammatical sentences are processed differently regardless of whether there is time pressure or not. In other words, it is the grammaticality that predicts the implicit/explicit distinction, not the timing of the response.

Not all researchers agree that (at least some kinds of) judgment data can tap into implicit knowledge. Vafaee, Suzuki, and Kachisnke (2017) challenge the notion that any kind of judgments—timed or untimed, on grammatical or ungrammatical sentences—can measure implicit knowledge. Their study consisted of responses by 79 Chinese learners of English on four different tests: 1) judgment tests (timed and untimed), 2) a self-paced reading task, 3) a word-monitoring task, and 4) a metalinguistic judgment task. Among the relevant findings for our purposes is the fact that the results from the self-paced reading task and the word-monitoring task (both online processing tasks that presumably tap into implicit knowledge) reflect a different construct than do the judgment tasks. Their general conclusion is that any type of judgment task draws attention to form and thereby draws on explicit knowledge. As they put it, judgment tasks "are too coarse to be measures of implicit knowledge" (p. 85).

Similarly, some researchers argue that judgment tasks, even timed ones, allow access to automatized explicit knowledge, that is, explicit knowledge that can be accessed quickly but is still available to conscious awareness (e.g., Suzuki & DeKeyser, 2015, 2017). Automatized explicit knowledge is thought to be distinct from implicit knowledge, which is knowledge without awareness. These researchers argue that judgment tasks cannot be used to measure implicit knowledge; instead, a better way to measure implicit knowledge is to measure reaction times and eye movements during the processing of meaning (e.g., comprehension tasks).

Indeed, some researchers use acceptability judgments with exactly the goal of measuring participants' explicit knowledge of grammar. For instance, Zufferey, Mak, Degand, and Sanders (2015) investigated English discourse connectors such as *if* and *while* with French- and Dutch-speaking learners. Learners completed an eye-tracking task in which they read sentences with correct and incorrect sentences and answered short comprehension questions. They also completed an untimed, written, paper-and-pencil acceptability judgment task with correct and incorrect use of discourse connectors. More negative transfer effects were found for the judgment task than for the online task. The authors interpret these results to mean that the learners' knowledge of discourse connectors is largely procedural and not easily accessible to conscious awareness. When learners access their explicit knowledge, they transfer patterns from the first language.

In summary, many researchers have used judgment data as one way of tapping into learners' knowledge of grammar. Some have targeted explicit knowledge, but many have also targeted implicit knowledge. There is evidence that judgment data can tap into implicit knowledge, in particular when judgment tasks are timed and when responses to grammatical stimuli are considered. However, doubts remain as to whether explicit knowledge plays a role in learners' judgments, even on timed grammatical stimuli. For this reason, it is probably wise to consider judgment data among other measures, such as elicited production data, ERP data, eye-tracking measures, and so on, in an effort to build a more complete picture of learners' abilities and knowledge.

2.5. What Are Judgment Tasks Used for?

In the previous section, we discussed judgment data as they relate to the measurement of explicit and implicit knowledge. However, judgment data have been used for a wide range of purposes, contexts, and subdomains. They have also been used for a range of research purposes, for example, to show development over time, to assess proficiency, to screen participants, and to determine knowledge types.

Based on the extensive survey in Plonsky et al. (in press) most judgment tasks measure static knowledge (89%) (e.g., Abrahamsson, 2012; Clahsen, Balkhair, Schutter, & Cunnings, 2013; Cox & Sanz, 2015; Zhang, 2015), and a few are used to determine development (11%) (e.g., Indrarathne & Kormos, 2017; Yalçin & Spada, 2016). Within the categories of static knowledge and development, other categories appear, such as the use of judgments to assess proficiency (e.g., Ayoun, 2014; Philp & Iwashita, 2013), to screen participants (Athanasopoulos, 2006), to understand the extent to which there is a critical or sensitive period for acquisition, and to determine knowledge types (e.g., Li, Ellis, & Zhu, 2016). In Chapter 3, we will provide a more detailed account of the frameworks and purposes that have seen judgment data as part of their data base.

2.6. Intervening Variables

Perhaps more so than native speaker judgments, L2 judgments are variable. It is important to weed out factors that may interfere. In fact, Schachter (1989) pointed out the need to distinguish between true judgments of acceptability and those where processing constraints intervene. In her article, she critiqued what at the time was a ground-breaking study by Ritchie (1978). Her point was that many of his sentences were actually garden-path sentences that were difficult for anyone (native or non-native) to process. In other words, a rejection of a sentence may have been due to processing difficulty, and the results were not a true reflection of the interlanguage grammar of the learner.

The concern about the effect of processing difficulty on judgments can be traced back to Chomsky (1957) and Chomsky and Miller (1963), who made a distinction between grammaticality and acceptability based on the idea that certain sentences that follow the principles of English grammar may still be rated as unacceptable because they are too difficult to process. For instance, consider sentences with multiply embedded relative clauses, as in Example 2:

Example 2. The soup that the chef that the restaurant manager hired prepared simmered.

Many speakers might rate this sentence as unacceptable because it is difficult to process, especially if they read it quickly.

Culicover (2013) argues that acceptability is related to complexity. If something is complex, unacceptability may arise. For example, certain structures, such as passive, may cause mild processing difficulty that could affect judgments. Consider the sentences in Example 3, specifically the use of the zero-relative clause marker (Ø) (from Culicover, p. 261). Culicover points out that the more syntactic complexity (because of the number of constituents and branching nodes) between the head of the noun phrase and the zero relative clause marker, the less acceptable the sentences become.

Example 3.
a. the decision [that/ Ø] you admit you regretted
b. the decision to attack [that/ Ø] you admit you regretted
c. the decision to attack while screaming [that/ ?Ø] you admit you regretted
d. the decision to attack the campground [that/ ?Ø] you admit you regretted
e. the decision to attack the campground without any warning [that/ ?Ø] you admit you regretted
f. the decision that you were going to attack the campground without any warning [that/ ?Ø] you admit you regretted
g. the decision revealed last night that you were going to attack the campground without any warning [that/ ??Ø] you admit you regretted

The question thus arises: how does one differentiate between unacceptability that arises from complexity and unacceptability that arises from ungrammaticality?

Fanselow, Schlesewsky, Cavar, and Kliegl (1999) tested exactly this idea when they examined subject-initial and object-initial embedded questions in German. Native speakers took longer to read object-initial clauses than subject-initial clauses, despite the fact that both are grammatical in German. Fanselow and Frisch (2006) point out that the effect can work in reverse, as well; that is, when intermediate processing steps have greater acceptability, participants may be more likely to rate a sentence as more acceptable, even if the overall sentence is not fully acceptable. For instance, consider sentences 4a and 4b (Fanselow & Frisch, 2006, pp. 15–16). As in English, German requires subject–verb agreement but does not have a clear verb form to use when two noun phrases are coordinated with *oder* 'or.' This issue arises both with verbs that overtly mark agreement (as in Example 4a) and with verbs that do not (as in Example 4b).

Example 4. a. er oder ich schlafe/schläft/schlafen

he or I sleep1sg sleep3sg sleep3pl

b. er oder ich darf schlafen

he or I may (no overt agr.) sleep

Fanselow and Frisch find that native-speaker participants rate 4b as more acceptable. They argue that the ambiguity in the verbal agreement in 4b influences participants' rating of the entire sentence, specifically, by improving its acceptability. Whether these processing issues would affect non-native judgments similarly is not known.

2.7. Conclusion

In this chapter, we have presented a background of some of the major issues confronting researchers as they use judgment data in second language research. In Chapter 3, we present an overview and provide examples of studies that have used judgment data within a variety of frameworks and to address a range of L2 research issues.

Notes

1. Additional criteria for inclusion were:

   a. Studies must have had a morphosyntactic target to be included (e.g., studies targeting pragmatic knowledge were excluded).
   b. Studies must have used the following terminology: grammaticality judgment task/acceptability judgment task/truth-value judgment task etc. for a task that targeted the participants' additional languages, not their L1 (e.g., L2, L3).
   c. Studies must have reported on unique participant samples or focus on a target structure that was not included in any sister studies.

   Exclusion criteria were studies:

   a. In which participants were asked to make a choice between two or more options (e.g., binary or multiple-choice tasks) unless they were asked to rate the different options on a scale (see discussion in Neubauer & Clahsen, 2009);
   b. Including tasks in which participants were required to determine if a pair of sentences matched;
   c. In which the main focus was not on judgments but rather on reading times, ERPs, etc.;
   d. In which 'grammaticality' or 'acceptability' did not occur alongside 'judg(e)ment' and either 'test' or 'task';
   e. We took into account the issues of self-labelling; if authors self-labelled as grammaticality judgment or acceptability judgment but the instrument did not meet our inclusion criteria, these were then considered on a case by case basis. If authors did not self-label as grammaticality judgment or acceptability judgment but the instrument did meet inclusion criteria, then studies were included.

2. This is somewhat oversimplified because many L2 research designs incorporate grammatical target language sentences as well as ungrammatical target language sentences. In most instances, however, the ungrammatical sentences are intended to reflect the learner's interlanguage (often used as a proxy for their native language), but that is only a result of the researcher's experience (often based on a reading of the literature).
3. Justifications are still found, albeit less frequently. For example, El-Ghazoly, in a 2013 dissertation, devotes approximately two and a half pages to a discussion of the viability of using judgment data.
4. The hypothetical example was probably not so hypothetical in that Selinker himself was an adult language learner of Hebrew!
5. This refers to a system where everything is interrelated. This is frequently attributed to Saussure, but this attribution is in question (Koerner, 1996/1997).
6. *Language Learning* was the target journal because of its unique focus on second language learning and the fact that it was the only journal that covered the time period that the authors were interested in.
7. This period of time was selected for their analysis because the scope of their paper was the influence of Selinker's 1972 paper on interlanguage.
8. Other articles in the first time period were largely pedagogical (40) or descriptive (24), whereas articles other than empirical work in the second time period were in testing (21) or were position papers (29), with 22 papers dealing with other topics.
9. The significant attention devoted to implicit/explicit knowledge in the L2 literature, with timed versus non-timed responses being a distinguishing factor, may in part explain the rise in the use of acceptability judgments in the past two decades, as reflected in Figure 2.7.

3

USES OF JUDGMENTS IN L2 RESEARCH

3.1. Introduction

Judgments have been used for a variety of purposes, in studies with a variety of theoretical frameworks, investigating a range of constructs, and focusing on different areas of language. In what follows, we provide examples of the range of studies that have used judgment tasks with second language learners. In the final sections of the chapter, we provide additional summary data about the languages investigated as well as issues related to defining proficiency levels in L2 research.

3.2. Frameworks

Nearly every L2 theoretical framework has at some point made use of judgment data. This section outlines theoretical frameworks and research orientations and examines the purposes that judgment data serve within each one. While it is clearly not the case that judgments are equally used in all frameworks, we use examples to illustrate the types of research questions that have been asked and the conclusions that have been drawn on the basis of judgment data. Where possible, we have included studies that have occurred within the past decade or even in the past few years.

3.2.1. Formal Approaches

The use of judgment data in research taking a formal approach is common. Formal approach research focuses on the formal structure of language, for instance, word order within negation, questions, or relative clauses. One way to investigate formal issues is to examine how the similarities or differences between features present in the L1 vs. L2 may affect L2 acquisition. An example of this approach comes from Cho and Slabakova (2017), who conducted research using the feature reassembly approach (Lardiere, 2008, 2009), which focuses on the contrast between the way grammatical features are expressed in the native language and the target language. Cho and Slabakova's (2017) study involved English- (n = 49) and Korean-speaking (n = 53) learners of Russian, as well as a control group of NSs of Russian (n = 56). The target of study was Russian indefinite determiners, specifically *kakoj-to* and *kakof-nibud'*. *Kakoj-to* has the features −definite, −referential, and +specific and is similar to the functional morphemes *some* in English and *eotteon* in Korean. However, *kakof-nibud'* has a constellation of features that is not lexicalized in English or Korean; that is, there is no determiner in English or Korean with this set of features. Cho and Slabakova used what they called a felicity judgment task to test for semantic knowledge of specificity and a grammaticality judgment task to determine learners' knowledge of the grammaticality of the determiners in grammatical contexts.

An ANOVA was conducted with Group (Russian NS, L1 English, L1 Korean) and Condition (*kakoj-to* [acceptable in +specific], *kakoj-nibud'* [unacceptable in +specific], *kakoj-to* [unacceptable in −specific], *kakoj-nibud'* [acceptable in −specific]). The findings suggest that the morpheme learners performed best with (*kakoj-to*) was the one that had a corresponding morpheme in the L1 with the same feature constellation (English = *some*, Korean = *eotteon*). When there is no correspondence between the "featural make-up" (p. 318) of the L2 morpheme and a particular lexical item in the L1, learning is delayed. The authors conclude that feature reassembly poses a challenge for L2 learners.

Borgonovo, Bruhn de Garavito, and Prévost (2015) investigated the acquisition of mood in a second language through an analysis of data at the interface of morphosyntax and semantics. Their particular focus was the Spanish subjunctive. They explored differences between the subjunctive in Example 1 (Borgonovo et al., 2015, p. 35):

Example 1. Busco unas tijeras que corten alambre

I look for scissors that cut- SUBJ wire

and the indicative in Example 2:

Example 2. Busco unas tijeras que cortan alambre

I look for scissors that cut- IND wire

Both are grammatical, but the indicative indicates that the speaker is looking for a specific pair of scissors, whereas the subjunctive has the meaning of "any pair of scissors" as long as they will cut. Two tests were administered, a judgment task and what the authors call an appropriateness judgment task. Thirty-eight English-speaking learners of Spanish were divided into two groups (based on two standardized tests of Spanish proficiency): intermediate and advanced. The acceptability judgment task was used as a preliminary filter to the appropriateness judgment task; in other words, it served to ensure that learners could distinguish between the subjunctive and indicative moods. Participants were asked to judge 24 sentences on a 5-point scale ranging from completely ungrammatical to completely grammatical. There was also an "I don't know" option, which they were told to avoid as much as possible.

The appropriateness judgment task consisted of 36 scenarios (see Examples 3 and 4) with two sentences following each (p. 50). They were asked to say whether each sentence was appropriate or not for the scenario, using the same scale as in the acceptability judgment task.

Example 3. It is Marisol's birthday. Her friends don't know what to get her, so they ask her boyfriend. He saw a perfume advertised on TV, and he knows she wants it. He says:

a. Marisol quiere un perfume que anuncien en la televisión.

M. wants a perfume that announce- SUBJ on the television.

b. Marisol quiere un perfume que anuncianen la televisión.

M. wants a perfume that announce- IND on the television.

Example 4. I must spend a week in a hotel, but I cannot leave my dog alone at home. The problem is that most hotels don't allow pets in the rooms. I ask a friend of mine:

a. ¿Conoces un hotel que acepte perros?

know-you a hotel that accept- SUBJ dogs

b. ¿Conoces un hotel que acepta perros?

know-you a hotel that accept- IND dogs

Results suggested that learners could distinguish between the appropriateness of the two moods, although learners were better at rejecting inappropriate subjunctives than inappropriate indicatives.

3.2.2. Usage-Based Approaches

In usage-based approaches, the argument is that learning takes place over time based on exposure to exemplars in the input. Memory traces from each exposure inform learners of frequency patterns in particular contexts, so that learners can make use of statistics to determine possible sentences. Learners take note of non-occurrences as well as occurrences, so that they can also determine sentences that are not possible (so-called indirect negative evidence). Robenalt and Goldberg (2016), in an extension of their 2015 study, compared native- and non-native-listeners' perceptions of the acceptability of ill-formed sentences based on the frequency of the verb utilized. Two sentence types were investigated, each featuring a high and low frequency verb (p. 69). In sentence Type A, the target sentence had a competing alternative (see Example 5 [alternative in parenthesis]). In Type B, there was no competing alternative formulation (see Example 6).

Example 5. High Frequency: Amber explained Zach the answer. (Amber explained the answer to Zach.)

Low Frequency: Amber recited Zach the answer. (Amber recited the answer to Zach.)

Example 6. High Frequency: Megan smiled her boyfriend out the front door.

Low Frequency: Megan grinned her boyfriend out the front door.

In the 2015 study, native English speakers provided lower acceptability ratings for sentences with high frequency verbs when there was a competitor. However, when no competitor was available, sentences with the two verb types were seen as equally acceptable. The authors interpreted this to indicate that native speakers are "highly sensitive to the presence of competing alternative phrasing. . . [but] when no competitor exists, speakers display a willingness to extend a verb to a construction in which it does not normally appear" (Robenalt & Goldberg, 2016, p. 69).

The 2016 study extended the 2015 findings by including the acceptability perceptions of L2 learners of English. Acceptability ratings (using a 5-point Likert scale) were elicited from 157 NSs and 276 adult L2 learners of English using Amazon's Mechanical Turk (www.mturk.com) (see Chapter 4, Section 4.2.13). Fourteen verb pairs (28 verbs total) were presented to learners in two sentence frames (typical usage, atypical usage), and acceptability ratings were analyzed using mixed-effects modeling. Whereas NSs maintained the pattern for verbs in atypical sentence frames found in Robenalt and Goldberg (2015), NNSs did not demonstrate an effect for competitor formation or frequency of verbs. However, an *a posteriori* consideration of non-native speaker proficiency did reveal that at higher proficiency, the participants' behavior began to align more closely with native speaker ratings. The authors interpreted their results as indicating that non-native speakers do not possess the ability to make necessary predictions. They learn primarily from positive exemplars and do not take alternative grammatical possibilities into account.

3.2.3. Skill Acquisition Theory

In skill acquisition theory, practice is seen as an important means to acquiring a second language. DeKeyser (2007) explains how the acquisition of knowledge occurs through a series of steps: "people are first presented with *information*, e.g., rules about how to . . . put a French sentence together in explicit form ('declarative knowledge')" (p. 3). The next step occurs when, through practice, this information turns into "*behavioral routines* ('production rules,' 'procedural knowledge')" (p. 3). Through practice, these "routines" become fast and virtually error free. Through continued practice, procedural knowledge becomes automatized, which, in

> the broadest sense . . . refers to the whole process of knowledge change from initial presentation of the rule in declarative format to the final stage of fully spontaneous, effortless, fast, and errorless use of that rule, often without being aware of it anymore.
>
> *(p. 3)*

Khatib and Nikouee (2012) used skill acquisition theory as the basis for their study, which specifically tests whether declarative knowledge can be automatized through practice. Their linguistic target was the English present perfect. They compared two groups of English as a foreign language learners (EFL learners), who both received instruction that included 1) rule explanation, 2) mechanical practice, and 3) meaningful practice. One group (group 1, n = 10) also received planned communicative practice; the other (n = 10) only received explanation and mechanical and meaningful practice. Knowledge was assessed by means of an untimed judgment test with four grammatical items, with eight additional items included as fillers. Even though participants could take as long as they needed, their response time was measured. Thus, the researchers were able to measure two aspects of automatization: decrease in errors and decrease in time. Following the treatment, follow-up testing was done two days later and two weeks later. At both times, the group that received communicative practice outperformed the group that did not.

3.2.4. Input Processing/Processing Instruction

Input processing is a theory of SLA that focuses on how learners make initial form-meaning connections (VanPatten & Williams, 2015). This includes how connections are made, why some connections are made and others are not, and the relationship between the acquisition process and the strategies employed by learners to comprehend input. Multiple principles have been proposed to describe how learners initially process incoming input (e.g., the first-noun principle and the primacy of content words; see VanPatten, 2012). An extension to input processing is processing instruction, which "teaches learners to process input differently than when they are left to their own devices" (Marsden, 2006, p. 313). Specifically, input processing pushes learners to interpret not only the meaning of a sentence but the linguistic forms within the input that create this meaning.

To compare the effects of explicit instruction versus explicit + processing instruction among young adult (n = 10) and older (n = 11) L1 English/L2 Spanish bilingual learners of Latin, Cox and Sanz (2015) utilized a 20-item (12 critical, 8 fillers) judgment test (as part of a 4-test battery) in a pre-, post-, and delayed posttest design. The judgment test targeted thematic role assignment (i.e., *patient* versus *agent* in transitive sentences). A separate grammar test on metalinguistic knowledge was included, administered after explicit instruction, but before processing instruction. The results showed overall gains by the two groups (young adults and older adults), but no difference between explicit instruction versus explicit + processing instruction. The authors reason that the judgment task prompts the use of an explicit rule (p. 242) and interpret the results to mean that providing processing on top of explicit instruction does not yield a lasting ability to explicitly judge acceptability.

3.2.5. Processability Theory

Processability theory (Pienemann, 1998, 2005) proposes that certain syntactic and morphological forms and structures emerge in a similar order for L2 learners, regardless of their first language. Empirical research into English, Japanese, Swedish, Italian, and Arabic (among others) has provided robust support for processability theory (Spinner, 2013). While the stages of processability theory have been altered and adapted over the years, the five key stages (listed in implicational order) are 1) lemma access, 2) category procedure, 3) phrasal procedure, 4) S-procedure, and 5) subordinate clause procedure. Whereas a large majority of processability theory research has been conducted through an analysis of L2 learner production, as will be described below, judgment tasks have more recently been utilized to take into account receptive knowledge.

As a means to further develop a model of interlanguage, Spinner (2013) investigated whether the implicational order predicted by processability theory for language production is similar to that which emerges for language reception. Three individual studies were conducted, each building on the results of the previous. In Study 1, 51 English NNSs (and 40 NSs) completed a 150-item acceptability judgment task targeting 15 structures across the five stages of the processability theory hierarchy. Each sentence was rated as "Correct" or "Incorrect" (with an "I don't know" option also provided). Through the use of implicational scaling (based on grammatical rating accuracy), results indicated that the predictions of processability theory for production did not predict the NNSs' performance on the judgment task.

After a subset of 12 speakers from Study 1 completed an interview in Study 2, it was confirmed that despite not adhering to processability theory for receptive knowledge, these NNSs provided nearly perfect implicational tables for productive knowledge. Based on the findings of Studies 1 and 2, Study 3 was conducted with a revised acceptability judgment task (based on item reliability) completed by

63 NNSs (and 15 NSs). As was found with Study 1, receptive knowledge did not align with the predictions of processability theory for productive development. From these findings, the author reasons that grammatical decoding (receptive knowledge) may operate somewhat autonomously from grammatical encoding (productive knowledge).

3.2.6. Interactionist Approaches

Interactionist approaches towards language acquisition stress the importance of input, interaction, feedback, and output, accounting for learning through learners' exposure to and production of the target language, along with feedback received on this production (Gass & Mackey, 2015). Within interactions, it is hypothesized that language learning is facilitated when there is a communication breakdown (e.g., Long, 1996). During these episodes, interlocutors are required to negotiate for meaning, with both NSs and NNSs performing discourse moves such as clarification requests or comprehension and confirmation checks. For learners, such breakdowns may provide negative evidence that signals a gap in their interlanguage, which in turn leads to noticing and, ideally, a reformulation of their interlanguage. One way in which this negative evidence may be presented is through corrective feedback, which has been the source of many empirical intervention studies, some of which have utilized judgment tasks to measure the effectiveness of different feedback techniques.

In a pre-, post-, and delayed posttest design, Li (2013) investigated the relationship between feedback type (either recasts or metalinguistic explanations) and learners' aptitude (specifically, language analytic ability and working memory). Seventy-eight L2 Chinese learners (L1 English [75], Korean [3]) were divided into three feedback groups: those who received recasts, those who received metalinguistic explanations, and a control. These groups completed a three-session procedure (pretest, treatment/posttest, delayed posttest) with a focus on Chinese classifiers. For each test period, learners completed an elicited imitation task and a 23-item acceptability judgment test (15 target, 8 filler). Learners either judged the acceptability of each item or indicated that they did not know. For each item marked ungrammatical, they were asked to locate and correct the error. Regression analyses were conducted on two sets of gain scores (between the pretest and the posttest, and the pretest and the delayed posttest) for both the elicited imitation and judgment tests. While all three groups showed improvement from pretest to posttests, the improvement was greatest for the metalinguistic group and smallest for the control group. The distance between the metalinguistic and recast groups after the delayed posttest was smaller than after the immediate posttest. In terms of aptitude, language analytic ability explained 20% of variance in judgment test gain scores for the recast group but was not a significant predictor for the metalinguistic group. Working memory accounted for 30% of variance in judgment test gain scores for the metalinguistic group ($p < .01$), but did not significantly predict performance for the recast group. Importantly, these findings were only for the delayed scores. The author interprets these findings as supporting the importance of further investigating the interaction between aptitude and treatment type (i.e., feedback), as "characteristics of each learning condition . . . set different processing demands on learners' cognitive abilities" (p. 649). That is, there are multiple dimensions in the relationships between aptitude and feedback type.

3.2.7. Sociocultural Theory

Sociocultural theory originates from the work of Vygotsky and colleagues and proposes that "developmental processes take place through participation in cultural, linguistic, and historically formed settings such as family life, peer group interaction, and in institutional contexts like schooling, organized social activities, and work places (to name only a few)" (Lantolf, Thorne, & Poehner, 2015, p. 207). A key component of sociocultural theory is that what can be accomplished working alone is not as great as what can be accomplished in collaboration with a more capable peer. The difference between these two is referred to as the Zone of Proximal Development (Vygotsky, 1978). When learners communicate socially, they appropriate patterns and meanings within social speech and utilize those patterns to mediate their own mental activity in private speech. Private speech is defined as "an individual's externalization of language for purposes of maintaining or regaining self-regulation, for example to aid in focusing attention, problem solving, orienting oneself to a task, to support memory related tasks, to facilitate internalization of novel or difficult information" (Lantolf et al., 2015, pp. 210–211).

Focusing on private speech as a source of self-regulation during L2 development, Stafford (2013) investigated the initial stages of L2 learning. Recruiting nine Spanish–English bilinguals, Stafford targeted the assignment of thematic roles in Latin, an unknown language to the participants. During a series of computer-moderated lessons, participants were asked to verbalize their thought process as they heard and saw a series of sentences, performed a task (picture choice, sentence translation), and received feedback. A 12-item acceptability judgment test was included in a four-test battery to assess learning outcomes, both immediately and after three weeks. Participants were asked to determine the acceptability of Latin sentences with a binary rating scale including an "I don't know" option. While the judgment test was only a part of the test battery, general results indicated that some learners were more successful than others. However, the amount of private speech did not seem to align directly with gains, as the two most successful learners demonstrated both the most and least private speech. In summarizing her finding, the author proposes that while some learners were able to enjoy success based on their own private speech, others were in need of a more direct, adaptive partner.

3.3. Knowledge Types

Beyond the theoretical approaches described above, in recent years, focus has turned to the use of judgment data to distinguish between knowledge types, primarily between implicit/explicit knowledge and procedural/declarative knowledge.

3.3.1. Implicit and Explicit Knowledge

The constructs of implicit and explicit knowledge hold a significant place in SLA research. At its simplest, explicit knowledge can be seen as knowledge learners can retrieve and are aware they possess, while implicit knowledge is unconscious, with learners unaware they possess it (Loewen, 2015). One key stream of explicit/implicit inquiry has been the validation of tools to measure these two knowledge types. Ellis (2005) and various studies since (e.g., Bowles, 2011; Zhang, 2015) have examined oral imitation, oral narration, metalinguistic knowledge tests, and both timed and untimed acceptability judgment tests. Specifically, in these studies it is hypothesized that timed acceptability judgment tasks measure implicit knowledge, while untimed acceptability judgment tasks measure explicit knowledge. The difference lies in time pressure, which appears to limit a learner's ability to reflect upon the knowledge they possess, requiring more use of intuition. Without time pressure, learners are able to search for explicit knowledge to make an accurate judgment.

3.3.2. Procedural/Declarative Knowledge

Procedural and declarative knowledge were discussed previously in reference to skill acquisition theory, where it is proposed that learners begin with knowledge they are aware they have (declarative) and move towards the ability to use this knowledge (procedural). Another way to conceptualize this knowledge is in the form of memory. Declarative memory includes knowledge of facts and events related to the world and self (Ullman, 2001). Learning declarative knowledge can occur quickly and with limited exposure, but it requires attentional resources such as working memory and usually the intent to learn (Knowlton & Moody, 2008). Procedural memory, in comparison, underlies both motor and cognition skill and relates to habit learning. In this case, learning generally occurs gradually with repeated exposure. It requires fewer attentional resources and generally occurs without intention (Knowlton & Moody, 2008; Ullman, 2001). Importantly, unlike declarative memory, procedural memory is not consciously available to learners.

Through having participants study an artificial L2 (Broncanto2), Morgan-Short, Faretta-Stutenberg, Brill-Schuetz, Carpenter, and Wong (2014) considered the role of procedural and declarative memory in learning an L2. Fourteen English-speaking participants completed four tests of procedural and declarative learning ability, then participated in four training sessions. Assessment of learning was carried out twice (after the initial and final training sessions) using a timed, auditory judgment task (120 items: 60 grammatical, 60 ungrammatical). Participants judged sentences as either "Good" or "Bad." Analysis was conducted using *d'* scores, which take into account potential response bias (i.e., tendency to answer in a particular way). A paired-samples *t*-test indicated a significant improvement in judgment task performance from time 1 to time 2. Two-tailed Pearson correlations indicated judgment task performance at time 1 correlated significantly with declarative learning ability but did not correlate with procedural learning ability. At time 2, the opposite was found; that is, performance correlated only with procedural learning ability. The findings support theoretical perspectives that propose declarative and procedural memory are predictive of individual L2 grammatical development.

3.4. Specific Constructs

Aside from the theoretical frameworks and conceptualizations of knowledge discussed above, judgment tasks have been employed as tools to investigate other areas of interest to SLA researchers.

3.4.1. Critical/Sensitive Period

It has been proposed that a language can only be fully developed if learned within the period between infancy and adolescence (Lenneberg, 1967). Whether such a critical period affects L2 development has been a point of inquiry and heated debate within the field of SLA (e.g., see Muñoz & Singleton, 2011; Singleton, 2001). In this debate, judgment tasks have played an important role. A well-known study in this area is Johnson and Newport (1989), who compared L1 Chinese and Korean learners of English with early ages of arrival (AOAs) (before 15; n = 23) to those with late AOAs (after 17; n = 23). A 276-item acceptability judgment test (140 grammatical, 136 ungrammatical) targeted 12 English grammatical structures. Analyses using correlations and *t*-tests indicated a clear and strong advantage for early AOA learners across all target structures. The authors interpreted these findings as support for the existence of a critical period for acquiring a second language. Johnson and Newport's study and stimuli have been the source of several replications and adaptations over the years (e.g., DeKeyser, 2000; DeKeyser, Alfi-Shabtay, & Ravid, 2010; Larson-Hall, 2008; Slavoff & Johnson, 1995).

3.4.2. Working Memory

The role of working memory in SLA has been of significant interest, with much discussion on the role it plays as an individual difference between learners (e.g., Mackey, Adams, Stafford, & Winke, 2010). Working memory "assumes that a limited capacity system, which temporarily maintains and stores information, supports human thought processes by providing an interface between perception, long-term memory and action" (Baddeley, 2003, p. 829). In cognitive psychology, a common measure of working memory has been the use of counting, operation, and reading span tests (Conway et al., 2005), in which learners are exposed to a series of stimuli. Their ability to retain this information while conducting another task is seen as a measure of working memory. For example, in a reading span task, participants might be exposed to a series of sentences, each of which is followed by a letter. They are asked to judge the sentence as "making sense" or not. At the end of each block of sentences, participants must try to recall the letters that followed each sentence.

In SLA, judgment tasks have played a role in some working memory research. For example, working memory in second language learners may be measured by having learners judge sentences while they perform a memory task. For example, Alptekin, Erçetin, and Özemir (2014), Miller (2015), and Stafford (2011) all had participants judge the acceptability of a set of sentences and then repeat the last word of each sentence judged.

This procedure was also used by Coughlin and Tremblay (2013) to measure working memory in L2 learners, using an untimed, 98-item acceptability judgment task that assessed 52 L1 English participants' knowledge of number agreement in French. Participants judged each sentence as acceptable or not and were asked to correct any sentence judged as not acceptable. Participants performed at ceiling on the judgment task, indicating they possessed explicit knowledge of number agreement dependencies. Further data collected through a self-paced reading task, however, indicated that participants with higher working memory showed more sensitivity to number agreement violations, as measured by longer reading times on those items. Thus, while most participants performed well on the untimed judgments, they demonstrated more variation in the online self-paced reading task. Some of this variation can be accounted for by working memory.

3.5. Additional Research Areas

3.5.1. Neurolinguistic Processing

Similarly to the way that judgment tasks have served as a support tool for measuring working memory, they have also served in the analysis of neurolinguistic processing. In such studies, which often employ tools such as functional magnetic resonance imaging (fMRI; e.g., Wartenburger et al., 2003; Yang & Li, 2012) or event-related brain potentials (ERPs, e.g., Hahne & Friederici, 2001; Mueller, Girgsdies, & Friederici, 2008), judgment tasks are often used to elicit a response that can be measured. For example, Hahne and Friederici (2001) compared the processing of 12 L1 Japanese learners of German to that of native speakers using an auditory, 240-item judgment task. Incorrect items included either a semantic or syntactic error. While all participants performed relatively accurately on the judgment task, a comparison of brain activity between the learners and the NSs demonstrated differences depending on error type and grammatical accuracy. For sentences with a semantic violation, processing was similar between NS and NNS, whereas it differed for sentences with a syntactic violation. Interestingly, the NNSs processed sentences with no violation somewhat similarly to how NSs processed sentences with syntactic violations. The authors discuss how these processing differences may arise.

3.5.2. Neurocognitive Disorders

Judgment tasks have also been used to help understand the effects of neurocognitive disorders, such as Alzheimer's (e.g., Gómez-Ruiz, Aguilar-Alonso, & Espasa, 2012) and Broca's Aphasia (e.g., Alexiadou & Stavrakaki, 2006), on L2/bilingual processing. The Bilingual Aphasia Test (BAT) is a battery of tests designed to "assess each of the languages of a bilingual or multilingual individual [with aphasia] in an equivalent way" (Paradis, 2011, p. 427). The primary goal is to determine which of two languages might be best preserved, in order to better understand which is more appropriate for verbal communication, and to determine therapy for areas in need of treatment (Paradis, 2011, p 428). The BAT features a 10-item acceptability judgment test, along with a 10-item semantic acceptability test, in which participants indicate "yes" or "no" to the acceptability of each item in both of a bilingual's languages. (For an example of the English BAT, see www.mcgill.ca/linguistics/files/linguistics/english_bat.pdf.) Gómez-Ruiz et al. (2012) used the BAT to assess 12 Catalan–Spanish bilingual patients with early Alzheimer's. Nine of the 12 grew up in a Catalan monolingual environment, with their first exposure to Spanish occurring between 3 and 5 years of age. The other three were simultaneous bilinguals. While performance in Catalan and Spanish varied across tests, performance on acceptability judgments was better when items contained errors based on L2 (Spanish) interference on their L1 (Catalan) rather than errors based on L1 interference on the L2. Patients also scored higher in their L2 Spanish for semantic acceptability judgments, although this difference was not deemed clinically important by the authors. Overall, the authors indicate that while the patients' processing of their two languages is more similar than different, it is possible that regression to the L1 will increase as their Alzheimer's progresses.

3.5.3. Pragmatics

While the majority of the previous examples have focused on syntactic and morphological knowledge or development, judgment tasks have also been adapted as a means to assess L2 learners' pragmatic knowledge. Pragmatics "addresses language use and is concerned with the appropriateness of utterances given specific situations, speakers, and content" (Bardovi-Harlig & Dörnyei, 1998, p. 233). The primary goal of judgment tasks in this area is generally to determine to what extent learners deem certain items to be acceptable responses to a given stimuli. For example, in a pragmatic intervention study, Takimoto (2008) targeted lexical/phrasal and syntactic downgraders (that is, something that weakens the force of a statement). Sixty Japanese-speaking learners of English were exposed to one of three instructional conditions and then responded to various pragmatics knowledge tests. One of these was a judgment test. Learners were provided with a context, followed by a series of potential responses. They then rated the acceptability of each response in relation to the preceding context on an 11-point scale. See Example 7 below for an example provided in Takimoto (p. 377).

Example 7. Professor King at your university is a famous psychologist. You are now reading one of Professor King's books and finding it very complicated. You would like to ask Professor King some questions about the book. Professor King does not know you and Professor King is extremely busy. However, you decide to go and ask Professor King to spare you some time for some questions. What would you ask Professor King?

a. I want to ask you some questions?
b. I was wondering if it would be possible to ask you some questions?
c. Could I possibly ask you some questions?

Responses were then scored based on NS responses to the same stimuli. Pre- to posttest comparisons indicated the pragmatic instruction across the three groups led to improved performance for the learners.

In a study designed to measure the perception of severity of syntactic versus pragmatic errors, Bardovi-Harlig and Dörnyei (1998) used video stimuli to elicit acceptability judgments from English language learners and teachers in both second and foreign language settings. Items included either a grammatical or pragmatic error. Participants were asked to first identify if a target moment in the video was appropriate/correct and, if they responded no, to rate the severity of the problem. Results demonstrated that learners in an EFL setting identified grammatical errors at a much higher rate (82.4%) than they did pragmatic errors (61.9%), whereas English as a Second Language (ESL) learners were better at identifying pragmatic errors (84.6%) than they were at identifying grammatical errors (54.5%). While both ESL and EFL teachers identified grammatical errors quite well (> 90%), the ESL teachers were stronger at identifying pragmatic errors than their EFL peers (90.7% vs. 79.2%). In terms of severity, EFL learners and teachers rated grammatical errors as more severe, whereas ESL learners and teachers rated pragmatic errors as more severe. The authors interpret their findings to indicate that there is a need for greater awareness-raising of pragmatics in EFL contexts.

3.6. What Languages Have Been Used?

In the summary data from Plonsky et al. (in press), it is clear that the range of languages included in research with judgments is limited (see Tables 3.1 and 3.2 below). Much of the research focuses on either the learning of English (50% of the studies) or the learning of a second language by L1 English speakers (25% of the studies). Other commonly investigated languages are Chinese (L2 = 4%, L1 = 10%), Spanish (L2 = 14%, L1 = 4%), and French (L2 = 9%, L1 = 4%). Many studies conduct research in ESL settings with mixed-L1 classrooms (11%) or compare the judgments of learners with different L1s (15%). Some compare the judgments of mono- versus bilingual speakers (4%).

Most studies were conducted in a foreign language setting (52%) as opposed to a second language setting (41%). Artificial languages (4%) and heritage languages (8%) have also been investigated.

TABLE 3.1 List of participant L1s across judgment task studies based on data used in Plonsky et al. (in press).

Language as L1	*Number of studies*
English	96
Chinese	37
Japanese	19
French	17
Spanish	14
Arabic	12
Korean	12
Dutch	7
German	7
Greek	4
Portuguese	4
Russian	4
Turkish	4
Bulgarian	3
Persian	3
Hungarian	2
Polish	2
Croatian	1
Czech	1
Hebrew	1
Italian	1
Malay	1
Sinhala	1
Mixed L1 groups	44
Bilingual	12
L1 not reported	6

TABLE 3.2 List of target languages across judgment task studies (Plonsky et al., in press).

Target Language	*Number of Studies*
English	191
Spanish	55
French	34
Chinese	16
Artificial language	15
German	11
Swedish	9
Italian	7
Portuguese	7
Japanese	6
Dutch	5
Greek	5
Korean	5
Latin	4
Russian	2
Arabic	2
British Sign Language	2
Samoan	2
Afrikaans	1
Bulgarian	1
Esperanto	1
Filipino	1
Hebrew	1
Turkish	1

3.7. Proficiency Levels

In a review article, Thomas (1994) named four common ways in which proficiency is reported in L2 studies, namely, impressionistic judgments in which no justification or description is given for a particular proficiency determination, institutional status (e.g., fifth-semester Italian), in-house measures of proficiency (e.g., a placement test), or standardized tests. Based on the Plonsky et al. (in press) survey, it is difficult to determine precisely the proficiency levels of learners who have participated in research with acceptability judgments, because many studies use vague criteria to determine proficiency levels (if any criteria are used at all). Only 17% of the studies in that survey justified claims about proficiency against some external measure. The concern about a lack of a standard is not unique to studies using judgment data but rather is endemic to the field at large. Of course, in many studies a detailed determination of proficiency is not essential to answer the research question. However, with a relatively small number of judgment studies using external measures (such as standardized tests) to justify proficiency labels, it makes it more difficult to understand how intuitional knowledge changes over time or how judgment data may be impacted by proficiency.

3.8. Conclusion

In this chapter, we have provided examples of studies spanning a range of types, topics, and purposes that have used judgment data. In the next chapter, we turn to specific design issues and present common practices in the field as well as recommendations for using judgment data.

4

A GUIDE TO USING JUDGMENT TASKS IN L2 RESEARCH

4.1. Introduction

In any type of research, it is crucial that the methodology be appropriate to address the research question(s) being asked; that is, a research tool must be effective at eliciting data that can be used to provide an answer to the research question. In addition to relevance and appropriateness, practicality must also be considered. For instance, an elicitation tool that is unworkably long or complicated, or that needs to be administered one-on-one by trained personnel, may make it difficult, if not impossible, to collect enough data for findings to be robust. The choice of methodology, then, lies at the intersection of these two concerns: appropriateness and practicality.

Judgment tasks have long been seen as a practical choice, for the following reasons (among others):

1. They are relatively easy to design.
2. They can be administered either electronically or in a simple paper-and-pencil format. Particularly with the latter option, no special equipment or training is needed. This means they can be used in virtually any setting, and even with large groups.
3. Interpreting judgment data is relatively straightforward and does not require sophisticated statistics, fine-grained measures of reaction times, and so on, although sophisticated statistics can be used, and reaction time data can be collected.
4. They can be used for a wide range of language domains. In particular, they can be used for virtually any morphosyntactic issue of interest and are extremely versatile.
5. Data can be collected online with electronic tools (e.g., using Qualtrics or Amazon Mechanical Turk [see Section 4.2.13 for additional discussion]).

Another important rationale for the use of judgment tasks is that they can target knowledge of sensitivity to grammatical issues that may be difficult or impossible to examine by other means of elicitation, such as elicited production tasks, picture-matching, and so on. For example, judgment tasks have been used extensively to investigate learners' sensitivity to subjacency violations in long-distance *wh*-movement, as in *What do you wonder who saw?* (e.g., Johnson & Newport, 1991; Schachter, 1989; Uziel, 1993; White & Juffs, 1998). Because long-distance *wh*-movement does not regularly occur in spontaneous speech production and is difficult to elicit in a natural way, it is unlikely that elicited production tasks would be effective at definitively demonstrating whether learners find sentences with subjacency violations acceptable. On the other hand, a judgment task provides clear and direct evidence regarding learners' responses to these types of errors, when compared with sentences that contain grammatical long-distance *wh*-movement (e.g., *Who do you believe Mary likes?*).

As with any research instrument, a decision to use that instrument is only the first step. Judgment tasks differ on a wide variety of features, and the choice of a particular design may affect the type of data that are elicited as well as the reliability of the results.

In the following sections, we outline the many considerations that must be taken into account when designing and administering a judgment task. Following each discussion, we include general recommendations and/or issues to consider. These recommendations are narrow in the sense that they are made without reference to any specific context. Like all research decisions, there are trade-offs. Ideal conditions often do not exist, and researchers find themselves forced to make choices based on practicality or availability of resources or participants. For these reasons, it is important to keep in mind that our recommendations are decontextualized and are made in the abstract, ignoring the other exigencies that necessarily come into play in all research decision-making. As an example, consider our first recommendation (Box 4.2) that the number of sentences should be between six and ten per grammatical element. This works well if there are only one or two grammatical elements. But what happens if there are many? How many is too many? A decision would have to be made regarding the need to have a sufficient amount of data for an appropriate statistical analysis versus burdening participants to such an extent that one no longer has confidence in their responses. Similarly, the extent to which participants may become fatigued due to the task length depends on many factors, including the age and maturity of the participants. In this case, factors other than the number of sentences per element have to be taken into account in a research design, resulting in a cascading effect with one decision impacting another.

Whatever decisions are ultimately made, piloting the study is essential. It is through piloting that revisions are made, giving the researcher confidence (and justification) for the ultimate form of the task.

4.2. Design Features

It is important to recognize the effect that design features can have on learner performance on judgments. In a study of 93 learners of English as a foreign language, Spada, Shiu, and Tomita (2015) considered many design features, such as modality (aural versus written), stimulus type (grammatical versus ungrammatical), and timing (untimed versus timed). An important conclusion from their study was that design features significantly impacted learner performance, but the particular linguistic structure under investigation did not.

4.2.1. Total Number of Sentences to Be Judged

In designing any judgment task, it is important to take into account the number of tokens necessary to produce a reliable result as well as the issue of how many sentences participants are asked to judge in one sitting. An important factor to consider in this regard is participant fatigue. That is, participants may lose the ability or desire to focus on the task after a certain number of judgments or a certain period of time. They may begin to guess or mark items at random, reducing the reliability of the measure. Therefore, a judgment task should not be too long. But how long is too long?

Some judgment tasks are quite short. For example, there are 23 total sentences in the judgment task used in Li (2013) and 26 sentences in the judgment task in Hwang and Lardiere (2013). On the other hand, many studies include more than 100 sentences, for instance, 150 (Spinner, 2013), 204 (Dekeyser et al., 2010), 240 (Batterink & Neville, 2013), 282 (Johnson & Newport, 1989), or 300 (Montrul, Davidson, De La Fuente, & Foote, 2014).

Cowan and Hatasa (1994) recommend a maximum of 60–72 sentences, while Gass and Mackey (2007) recommend between 50 and 60, although in neither case is there a rationale for this specific number. For this reason, these recommendations should be seen only as guidelines. If judgments on a large number of sentences are needed, there are ways to reduce the effects of participant fatigue. One option is to provide frequent breaks. For instance, Spinner (2013) provided a brief break after every 25 sentences and a longer one halfway through (after 75 sentences). Johnson and Newport (1989) told participants that they could pause anytime they felt tired. Another option is to reduce the number of grammatical structures being analyzed, possibly by breaking them down into a number of smaller experiments. Alternatively, it may be necessary to reduce the number of tokens per grammatical structure (see discussion in Section 4.2.2). If the number of tokens is reduced to under six per grammatical target, it might be wise to create multiple versions of the task, with groups of participants (who have been determined to be similar with a measure other than the judgment task itself) responding to a subset of the tokens for each structure. For instance, if there are six grammatical sentences examining the use of past tense and six ungrammatical sentences, they could be divided into two versions of the test with three grammatical and three ungrammatical sentences each. Conroy and Cupples (2010) took such an approach when investigating non-native versus native preferences for what they call *modal perfect* structures such as *you should have studied more.* They devised 24 lexical-*have* sentences (*He could have work at the shoe factory*) and 24 analogous sentences with modal perfect (*He could have worked at the shoe factory*), but divided them into two lists (12 and 12 each), and supplemented these lists with 52 filler and practice items (total = 76). Participants only responded to one of the two lists.

BOX 4.1 TOTAL NUMBER OF SENTENCES TO BE JUDGED

- Between 50 and 70 judgments can likely be done at one time without fatigue, although the specific number depends on the participants (e.g., age, proficiency level) and the type of judgments.
- If necessary, create time for breaks, or create two different tests and give them to two comparable groups.

4.2.2. Number of Grammatical and Ungrammatical Tokens per Grammatical Form/Structure

Because of differences in research purposes, there can be a wide range of tokens per grammatical form or structure being investigated. Researchers who investigate general proficiency in a second language have included only a few representative sentences for each of a wide range of grammatical targets, focusing on participants' overall performance rather than on a particular grammar issue. As an example, consider Ellis (2005), who examined 17 different grammatical structures with only four sentences to be judged for each one, including both grammatical and ungrammatical sentences. Typically, however, researchers who investigate more specific grammatical issues use a higher number of sentences for each grammatical feature, for at least the following reasons. First, participants may reject any particular sentence for reasons unrelated to the targeted item (see discussion in Section 4.2.10 regarding corrections). Second, there may be something about the particular lexical items or constructions in a given target sentence that influences the way learners respond to it. Using several sentences to get at a single target element improves confidence in the results.

Importantly, most researchers include an equal number of corresponding ungrammatical items for each grammatical item. For example, if a researcher is examining the appropriate use of past tense marking on verbs, both grammatical sentences (with the appropriate use of target language past tense marking) and ungrammatical sentences (with missing or incorrect past tense marking) are included. Both are needed to provide a full account of learners' knowledge regarding past tense marking. Even in cases where responses to ungrammatical items is not part of an analysis, it is generally a good idea to include them. For instance, in Spinner (2013), one goal was to determine the nature of learners' responses to sentences with adverbs first, such as *Yesterday we saw an eagle.* In this case, the interest centered on the acceptance of the sentence, not on the rejection of an alternative. Despite this fact, it was considered important to have an ungrammatical counterpart in order to ascertain whether learners genuinely accepted the sentences with adverbs first, or if they were simply biased towards a "yes" response to this type of structure when they were uncertain. It was difficult to find appropriate ungrammatical counterparts to the grammatical sentences, since adverbs can appear in a variety of locations. Ultimately, the sentences that were included had the following word order: *We saw yesterday an eagle.* Responses to these ungrammatical structures were not used to answer the research question, which consisted of determining the extent to which well-established procedures for production (within processability theory) are shared by the receptive system, but were instead examined for evidence of a response bias (i.e., a tendency to answer "yes" to all judgments). See Section 4.2.5 for more information on grammatical and ungrammatical pairs.

Most researchers use between six and ten sentences per grammatical element being examined. That is, most judgment tasks include three to five ungrammatical sentences for each grammatical structure, balanced by three to five grammatical sentences. Eight sentences per condition (four grammatical, four ungrammatical) is fairly common for studies in which judgment data are analyzed without being combined with other measures. Studies that include reading time or online measures such as self-paced reading or eye-tracking in addition to judgment data typically have higher numbers of sentences per condition, in line with recommendations for self-paced reading studies, which typically have 8 to 12 sentences or more per condition (see Jegerski & VanPatten, 2014).

Often the sentences examining a particular structure will be similar, differing mainly in the specific lexical items included (e.g., Kweon & Bley-Vroman, 2011). Sometimes, however, there is more variation. For instance, Hwang and Lardiere (2013) examined *-tul* plural marking in Korean with 13 target sentences. The 13 sentences comprised two or three sentences for each of six different types of grammatical errors with *-tul.*

BOX 4.2 NUMBER OF SENTENCES PER GRAMMATICAL ITEM

- Include between six and ten sentences for each specific grammatical element you want to examine, keeping in mind an appropriate overall length.

- Higher numbers of sentences per targeted grammatical element will lead to greater confidence in the results, but keep in mind possible participant fatigue.
- Balance the number of grammatical and ungrammatical sentences so that there are three to five grammatical sentences and three to five ungrammatical sentences for each element you want to examine.
- If judgments are combined with self-paced reading or eye-tracking methodologies, follow recommendations for those methodologies by including more sentences per condition.

4.2.3. Target and Non-Target Stimuli

In addition to the target grammatical and ungrammatical items that will provide the data for analysis, it is generally desirable to include sentences that are not related to the research question. These sentences are called fillers and distractors. There are several reasons for including these sentences. First, if participants see too many of the same kind of sentences, particularly when a certain structure is ungrammatical, they may figure out the goal of the study. This is usually to be avoided, because learners may change their response based on what they believe the researcher is looking for. Second, if the sentences appear too similar, learners may adopt a strategy, such as paying attention only to certain parts of the sentence or applying a learned rule to each case. Finally, non-target sentences are intended to prevent structural priming effects, which refers to the phenomenon that participants are more likely to produce or comprehend a structure that they have recently heard. This effect might interfere with results.

It is important to note at this point that in some cases, researchers may not be concerned with many of these issues. For instance, Mai and Yuan (2016) investigated the acquisition of the *shi . . . de* construction in Chinese by native speakers of English. Specifically, the researchers wanted to know whether learners knew that the *shi . . . de* construction involves features [telic], [past] and [given]. Mai and Yuan used a judgment task along with other tasks to investigate learners' knowledge of this structure. Because instruction in the Chinese language rarely addresses these particular features, the researchers did not try to hide the goal of the study by using fillers and distractors. That is, the assumption was that learners did not have explicit knowledge to apply to the construction. Many failed to perform in a native-like manner, and the judgment task results paralleled results of other tasks. This example illustrates that judgment task design depends on the nature of the research goals and the linguistic target. Another case where researchers may not include fillers is with studies in which multiple grammatical elements are being examined. In this case, researchers may choose not to include any fillers because the stimuli are already quite varied; thus, the sentences examining different grammatical elements can serve as fillers for each other (see e.g., Granena, 2014; Johnson & Newport, 1989).

For studies in which fillers are used, there are often an equal number of target and filler items (e.g., Marsden & Chen, 2011). Some follow recommendations from quantitative psychological research (see, for example, Sagarra & Herschensohn, 2011) and include about twice as many fillers as target sentences (or more), so that at least two thirds of the stimuli are fillers.

Bordag and Pechmann (2007), in a study of gender retrieval by L1 Czech speakers learning German, presented data from four different experiments. In one experiment, 48 noun phrases (consisting of a demonstrative pronoun plus a noun) were included, all mismatched for noun gender and demonstrative pronoun. The demonstrative pronoun forms corresponded to what one might predict from the noun ending; in other words, nouns with typically feminine endings (e.g., Käse 'cheese'), but which were in actuality masculine, were paired with feminine demonstrative pronouns (*diese [f] Käse [m]). In this study, there were 48 noun-demonstrative pronoun pairs that were incongruent. In addition, there were 36 grammatically incorrect filler phrases and 84 grammatically correct noun phrases. Thus, in total, there were 168 items, of which 48 were the target items with 120 fillers (grammatically incorrect phrases/correct noun phrases). Ten practice items were also included.

While there is no agreed-upon way to determine the best number of fillers for a judgment task, it is important to keep in mind item placement; researchers typically avoid having two or more of the same type of sentence appear next to each other. For example, a participant will never see two sentences that target the same kind of past tense marking in a row. To avoid this, stimuli are often "pseudorandomized," which means that they are initially randomized but small changes in the order are made post-randomization to avoid having the same kind of target structures appear consecutively (see Section 4.2.6). If an adequate number of fillers is used, it is easier to create a judgment task that does not fall into a predictable pattern or allow too many of the same types of errors in a row. To some extent, though, the number of fillers a researcher uses will depend on the type of response they intend to elicit, an issue that is discussed further below.

The creation of non-target stimuli requires some care. They should be similar enough to the target sentences so that they cannot easily be distinguished as fillers. For instance, they should not be noticeably longer or shorter, more or less complex. Similarly, it is frequently desirable that some non-target sentences include ungrammaticalities that are not related to the research question. If the target sentences are the only ones with ungrammaticalities, and learners detect these ungrammaticalities, learners may be clued in to the purpose of the study. However, it is not necessary to include an exactly equal number of ungrammatical fillers, as long as a some are present (see discussion above regarding the Bordag and Pechmann (2007) study).

BOX 4.3 TARGET AND NON-TARGET STIMULI

- It is generally wise to avoid making the grammatical target obvious. This can be done easily when multiple structures are being investigated. One serves to draw attention away from the others.
- If only a few structures are targeted, other unrelated sentences (fillers) should usually be added. Generally, some of these fillers should also be ungrammatical so that if a learner detects the error, the object of the study is not immediately apparent.
- Regardless of which option is selected, some sort of randomization is desirable (see Section 4.2.6).

4.2.4. Instructions and Practice Items

It can be easy to forget that providing judgments is a learned skill. Many participants may accept ungrammatical sentences if they can figure out what the intended meaning is, or they may reject grammatical sentences if they disagree with the statement or find it odd for any number of reasons. Therefore, providing careful instructions and practice items is an essential part of the process.

Researchers have struggled to provide participants with instructions that both are clear and concise and elicit judgments that truly depend on the grammatical acceptability of the sentences in question. In Table 4.1 is a sampling of terms that have been used as a way of describing to participants what it means to make an acceptable versus an unacceptable judgment. Finding the right wording is tricky, because researchers are often hoping to get learners to judge syntactic acceptability (and not, for instance, semantics), but they are also hoping that learners will avoid applying a metalinguistic rule that they have learned in class or from a text. These latter possibilities do not appropriately represent their own intuitions.

The exact wording used may also depend on the grammatical issue being targeted as well as the target audience. For instance, Inagaki (2001) investigated

TABLE 4.1 Descriptors provided for participants for judgment tasks.

Hawkins (1987)	"(not) expressed in good English"
Hulk (1991)	"good" or "bad"
Bardovi-Harlig and Dörnyei (1998)	"appropriate" or "not appropriate"
Inagaki (2001)	whether each sentence "sounds natural"
Lozano (2002)	"right" or "wrong"
Cook (2003)	"ok" or "not ok"
Bautista (2004)	"correct" or "incorrect"
Toth (2006)	"possible" or "impossible"
Bruhn de Garavito and Valenzuela (2008)	"acceptable" or "unacceptable"
Cuza (2013)	"odd" or "fine"

motion verbs with goal postpositional phrases, such as the following: *Sam went into the house* or *Sam walked into the house* versus sentences such as *Sam entered the house by walking* or *Sam went into the house by walking* (p. 163). It may be difficult to determine whether any of these sentences fits the description "ungrammatical," so Inagaki asked participants to rate them as "natural" or not. On the other hand, a judgment task that targets whether pronouns correctly agree in gender with their antecedent is more likely to use terms such as "grammatical" or "correct" (e.g., Sabourin, Stowe, & de Haan, 2006).

While some researchers provide fairly minimal instructions, others are more explicit. Below are instructions from several studies.

Instructions From Toth (2006)—available on IRIS [www.iris-database.org/]

On the following pages is a list of sentences. I want you to concentrate on how you feel about these sentences. Native speakers of Spanish often have different intuitions about such sentences, and there are no right or wrong answers. I want you to tell me for each one whether you think it sounds possible or impossible in Spanish. Read each sentence carefully before you answer. Think of the sentences as spoken Spanish and judge them accordingly. After each sentence you will see 7 numbers. For each sentence write only ONE of the numbers on the separate answer sheet provided to show what you think of the sentence. Do not go back and change your answers.

Note that the instructions direct participants to rely on how they "feel" about each sentence. They also specifically request that participants not go back to change their answers, presumably because learners may start to apply learned rules if they take time to think about them or figure out what the task is targeting. On a computer-delivered task, this can be easily done by presenting only one sentence at a time; on a paper and pencil task, participants can be provided with pens so that crossouts are obvious. Additionally, the first answer that comes to mind is generally seen as more representative of implicit knowledge than answers arrived at after longer consideration (Rebuschat, 2013). Bley-Vroman, Felix, and Ioup (1988), in one of the most thorough examples of instructions, provide even more detailed instructions that include example items.

Instructions From Bley-Vroman et al. (1988, p. 32)

Speakers of a language seem to develop a 'feel' for what is a possible sentence, even in the many cases where they have never been taught any particular rule.

For example, in Korean you may feel that sentences 1–3 below sound like possible Korean sentences, while sentence 4 doesn't. [The sentences below were actually presented in Korean.]

1) Young Hee's eyes are big.
2) Young Hee has big eyes.
3) Young Hee's book is big.
4) Young Hee has a big book.

Although sentences 2 and 4 are of the same structure, one can judge without depending on any rule that sentence 4 is impossible in Korean.

Likewise, in English, you might feel that the first sentence below sounds like it is a possible English sentence, while the second one does not.

1) John is likely to win the race.
2) John is probably to win the race.

On the following pages is a list of sentences. We want you to tell us for each one whether you think it sounds possible in English. Even native speakers have different intuitions about what is possible. Therefore, these sentences cannot serve the purpose of establishing one's level of proficiency in English. We want you to concentrate on how you feel about these sentences.

For the following sentences please tell us whether you feel they sound like *possible* sentences of English for you, or whether they sound like *impossible* English sentences for you. Perhaps you have no clear feeling for whether they are possible or not. In this case mark *not sure.*

Read each sentence carefully before you answer. Concentrate on the structure of the sentence. Ignore any problems with spelling, punctuation, etc. Please mark only one answer for each sentence. Make sure you have answered all 32 questions.

Note that the authors specifically discourage participants from focusing on spelling or punctuation issues, presumably to prevent them from searching for minor errors or typos. Instructions are often given in the target language, but with lower-proficiency groups it may be necessary to provide instructions in the native language so that participants are not confused about the nature of the task.

While these explicit instructions are useful for guiding participants to focus on the features of interest, most researchers use shorter instructions. For example, Spada et al. (2015—available on IRIS [www.iris-database/org/]) provide these instructions.

Instructions From Spada et al. (2015)—available on IRIS [www.iris-database/org/]

You are going to hear some English sentences. After you hear each sentence, you will be asked whether the sentence is grammatically Correct or Incorrect. Mark your answer on the sheet of paper. If you think the sentence is grammatically correct, put a check (✓) beside Correct, and if it is grammatically incorrect put a check beside Incorrect. If you are not sure, check Not sure.

Researchers often rely on practice items to give participants a sense of what they are looking for. Sometimes the practice items are accompanied by the expected answer, so that learners can observe that grammatical errors are the target, rather than semantic issues (Spinner, 2013; Zhang, 2015). For example, in Spinner (2013, experimental materials), practice items were as follows: *The apple red is nice* (ungrammatical), *The yellow car is very pretty* (grammatical), *John Mary likes a lot* (ungrammatical), and *My friend likes you a lot* (grammatical).

It is generally inadvisable to provide examples with the feature under investigation, since it will clue participants in to the answer the researcher is expecting. For this reason, practice items typically involve structures that are unrelated to the target grammatical feature. For example, Akakura (2012) investigated L2 English learners' judgments of English article usage. Each sentence had an underlined region to be judged. However, in the two practice sentences, neither underlined region contained an article ("We hope you will *enjoying* visiting Paris"; "I went to a flower shop. There were many *flower* in the shop window," p. 34).

About three to six practice items are typically given. Feedback on the accuracy of participants' responses are generally provided for the practice items (but not, of course, for the items in the actual judgment task). Participants should have a chance to ask questions after having seen the practice items; however, questions can be difficult to answer. For instance, if a learner asks, "What should I focus on?," the researcher must try to emphasize that the participant should simply do their best to decide whether each sentence sounds right to them, being consistent with the language in the instructions. Researchers may want to note that it is not possible to fail at a judgment task.

BOX 4.4 INSTRUCTIONS

- Be as precise as possible so that participants understand what they are to do; for instance, make sure they know not to focus on semantics, unless that is the goal of your study.
- Consider the population that you are dealing with and the potential need to have instructions translated (along with examples) into their native language.

- Provide about three to six practice items, more if necessary to make the task clear. Include both grammatical and ungrammatical items in your examples.
- Allow time for questions following the instructions.

4.2.5. Constructing Grammatical and Ungrammatical Pairs

Typically, researchers pair ungrammatical items with corresponding grammatical items so that a comparison can be made between the ratings on each. Ideally, the sentences will be identical except for the point of ungrammaticality, so that it is certain that no other aspects of the sentence, such as word choice, is the source of differences between ratings on grammatical and ungrammatical sentences. This means that each sentence will have a grammatical version and an ungrammatical counterpart, for example: *yesterday Mary ate some pizza* and *yesterday Mary eat some pizza*. However, when pairs of sentences like these are used, another problem is introduced: participants are likely to notice the repetition and the contrast between the two sentences and could use that information to develop strategies for completing the task. There are a number of ways to avoid this problem. Ideally, two versions of the judgment task are prepared. Each version has one member of the sentence pair: either the grammatical or the ungrammatical member, and each version also has an equal number of corresponding grammatical and ungrammatical items. These are then given to two comparable groups.

If creating two versions of the task is impractical or problematic, it is generally advised to use grammatical and ungrammatical counterparts that are very similar, but not identical (e.g., rather than *yesterday Mary eat the pasta* and *yesterday Mary ate the pasta*, use sentences such as *yesterday Mary eat the pasta* and *yesterday Susan ate the pizza*). Additionally, it is important to make sure that any possible intervening variables (such as frequency and plausibility of particular constructions, regular and irregular forms, and so on) are carefully balanced between the grammatical and ungrammatical items or between different conditions. If there are a large number of sentences with significant spacing between similar sentences, the problem is not likely to be of serious concern. Additionally, if data collection is done on a computer, with sentences disappearing from the screen following each response, the problem is less likely to be severe.

BOX 4.5 GRAMMATICAL AND UNGRAMMATICAL PAIRS

- When possible, create two versions of the judgment task with half the grammatical and ungrammatical items in each, and administer to comparable groups.

- If it is not possible to have two versions of the judgment task, create grammatical/ungrammatical pairs that are similar but not identical. Create distance between them in the task.

4.2.6. Randomization

It is typical to introduce items in a random order to prevent ordering effects. Ordering effects occur when some stimuli are responded to differently because they are at the beginning of the task (when learners are fresh, but also still figuring out how the task works), the middle, or the end (when learners are used to the task but possibly also bored, tired, or trying to finish quickly). In principle, it is best for sentences in acceptability judgments to be presented in a truly random order that is different for each participant. This can be accomplished easily with a number of software packages (such as E-prime [https://pstnet.com/welcome-to-e-prime-3-0/] or Superlab [www.cedrus.com/superlab/]), the availability of which likely accounts for the increase in individually randomized tests during the past 20 years.

One problem with using automatic randomization, however, is that several of the same type of sentence can appear in a row, possibly clueing the learner in to the purpose of the experiment or allowing them to develop a strategy for completing the task. As mentioned in Section 4.2.3, many researchers opt instead for pseudorandomization, in which the presentation of stimuli is unpredictable, but items of the same type are not allowed to cluster in groups of two or three (or more), and items of various types are scattered throughout the entire task. While ordering effects are minimized with pseudorandomization, they are still possible, so many researchers create two or more pseudorandomized orders to avoid having certain stimuli always appear first. A common approach is to use one order and then simply to reverse it for a second order (e.g., Marsden, 2008). Another approach that captures the "best of both worlds" for computer-administered judgment tasks is to put pseudorandomized stimuli into blocks with equal numbers of each type of item and then to randomize the order of the blocks.

Randomization is more difficult to accomplish with tasks that are not presented with a computer, but ordering effects can be lessened by creating several versions of the task to be used with groups of participants.

BOX 4.6 RANDOMIZATION

- If there is little concern regarding similar items giving away the goal of the study, randomize sentences by participant.
- If there is concern regarding accidental clustering of particular item types with a fully randomized design, create blocks of stimuli with

pseudorandomized equal distribution of item types, then randomize the blocks.

- If paper and pencil tests are used, create several versions so that items do not appear in the same order for each participant.

4.2.7. Ratings and Scales

There are many ways to structure participants' responses to a judgment task. One possibility is to allow for only dichotomous or binary judgments: that is, each sentence is judged to be either correct or incorrect. This was the approach favored by a number of early judgment tasks, such as Ard and Gass (1987), Johnson and Newport (1989), and Trahey and White (1993).[1] Dichotomous scales are still used in recent research, as well; it should be noted that they are very quick and simple and therefore may be preferred for certain situations, such as with very low-level learners, or with an audio judgment task where decisions must be made quickly. Often when a binary good/bad decision is asked, a third option is provided: *I'm not sure* or *I don't know* (e.g., Li, 2013). This option is provided in an attempt to minimize guessing if participants don't have a strong feeling about grammaticality. However, it may be the case that this option is not typically chosen by participants (see Ellis, 1991; Spinner, 2013), so there are doubts about its effectiveness at reducing guessing. If source ratings are provided (see Section 4.2.9), it may be unnecessary to include an *I don't know* option, since learners are asked to indicate when they are making guesses.

Another option is to use a Likert scale with more than two or three possible responses. The reason to include more than a binary choice is that speakers of a language, whether native or non-native, often perceive there to be a continuum of ungrammaticality (see Sorace & Keller, 2005; Duffield, 2004 for discussion; see also the discussion in Chapter 1 of this book on linguistic gradience). For example, *she recommended me a good restaurant* may sound strange, but not as unacceptable as *she described me a good restaurant*. A binary scale cannot capture this distinction. An example of a study that uses a Likert scale is Bruhn de Garavito's (2011), which examined subjects and objects in L2 Spanish using a 5-point scale. The author found that the various types of ungrammatical sentences were perceived by both native and non-native speakers as having differing levels of unacceptability. Some types were perceived as highly ungrammatical, with mean scores around 1, while others had ratings around the middle of the scale but lower than the grammatical sentences. It may be wise to use Likert scales even in cases where a straightforward "up or down" decision is expected. In these cases, a Likert scale may be more effective at capturing learners' ambivalence or uncertainty regarding certain structures.

If a Likert scale is used, there are a number of considerations regarding its design. The first issue is the number of points on the scale that will accurately and reliably capture participants' intuitions about grammaticality. In SLA judgment tasks, rating scales typically range from 4 to 7 points and only rarely go higher. However, the optimal number of points on a Likert scale has been considered at great length in educational measurement research, where scales of between 7 to 11 points are recommended to increase the reliability of the measure (see Winke 2014 for discussion). This research suggests that a scale with a higher number of response options may be preferable to the smaller scales that are typically used with judgment tasks.

A related issue is whether there are an even or odd number of points on the scale. An odd number of points leaves a middle point: for example, a 3 on a 1 to 5 scale, or a 0 on a scale from −3 to 3. It is not clear what this middle point indicates. It might be interpreted as a sentence that is neither truly grammatical nor truly ungrammatical, something a speaker might consider "okay, but not great." On the other hand, it may end up being chosen when participants have no clear sense of grammaticality but still need to provide a response. Sometimes, the middle point on the scale is given a label such as *I don't know*, but this is problematic in that it eliminates the possibility of a response that is truly midway between grammatical and ungrammatical—that is, a response that indicates *I am sure that this is halfway between grammatical and ungrammatical*—as opposed to *I don't really have a sense of whether this sentence is grammatical or ungrammatical*. For this reason, some researchers provide an odd scale but also include a separate *I don't know* option (e.g., Toth, 2008). For instance, Marsden (2008) used the scale shown in Figure 4.1. She used the phrase "Can't decide" for her *I don't know* option and separated it physically from the rest of the scale. Participants saw a picture with a question and an answer and were then asked if the answer is possible.

Another possibility is to discard the center responses entirely and not include them in the analysis (e.g., Montrul, Dias, & Santos, 2011), but this, of course, removes valuable data. Some researchers collapse the higher and lower end of the scale into dichotomous data, but we do not generally recommend this practice unless it is presented alongside mean data (see Chapter 6 for more information on analyzing scalar data).

Using an even number of points on the scale eliminates the middle point. This means that participants are forced to indicate that a sentence is grammatical or ungrammatical. Using an even-numbered scale with the addition of an *I don't know* option is an attempt to avoid the necessity of interpreting or throwing out ambiguous responses, but of course it forces participants to rate a sentence as at least somewhat grammatical or ungrammatical even if they feel that it is exactly in the middle.

An additional consideration is how to label the points on the scale. There are two main options: starting at 0 or 1 and going up (e.g., 1, 2, 3, 4) or starting at a negative number and moving up to positive numbers (e.g., −2, −1, 0, 1, 2). This is not a trivial issue; research suggests that the labeling of data points affects how participants respond (Hartley & Betts, 2010). In particular, a rating scale that ranges

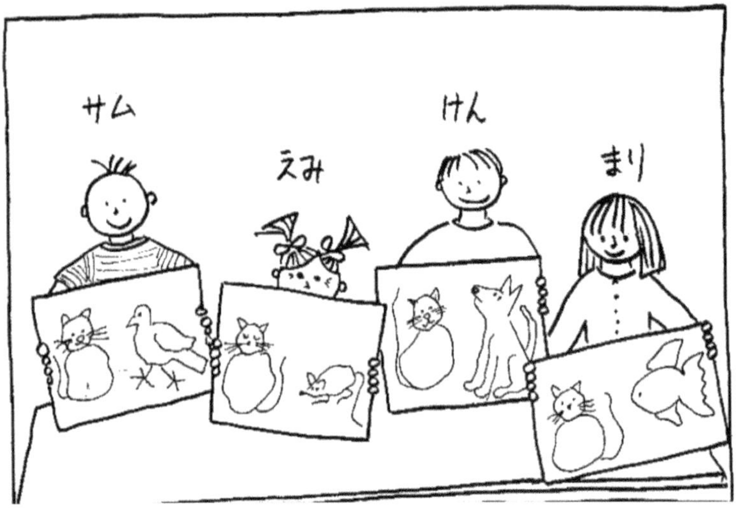

Q:	Nani-o	daremo-ga	kaita	no?
	what-Acc	everyone-Nom	drew	Q

'What did everyone draw?'

A:	Samu-kun-wa	neko	to	tori-o,	Emi-tyan-wa	neko	to	nezumi-o,
	Sam-*kun*-Top	cat	and	bird-Acc,	Emi-*tyan*-Top	cat	and	mouse-Acc,
	Ken-kun-wa	neko	to	inu-o,	Mari-tyan-wa	neko	to	kingyo-o
	Ken-*kun*-Top	cat	and	dog-Acc,	Mari-*tyan*-Top	cat	and	goldfish-Acc
	kaita.							
	drew							

'Sam drew a cat and a bird, Emi drew a cat and a mouse, Ken drew a cat and a dog, and Mari drew a cat and a goldfish.'

FIGURE 4.1A Response sheet to the question: Is the answer possible?

(Is the answer possible?)

	No, definitely not			*Yes, perfectly*	*Can't decide*
1	–2	–1	+1	+2	x
2	–2	–1	+1	+2	x

FIGURE 4.1B Pair-list answer test item and answer sheet

Source: From "Pair-list readings in Korean-Japanese, Chinese-Japanese and English-Japanese interlanguage" by E. Marsden, 2008, *Second Language Research*, *24*, p. 203, by Sage Journals. Reprinted by permission.

from negative to positive numbers reinforces the notion of ungrammaticality for sentences receiving negative numbers and provides a clear distinction between ungrammatical and grammatical sentences. A scale with all positive points may give the impression that grammaticality is a bit more fluid.

Other scales use descriptors for the rating points, either with or without numbers. Descriptors are varied, as noted earlier in the discussion about instructions (see Section 4.2.4). In Table 4.2, we present examples of scales used in judgment studies.

Most studies include some variant of the scale used in Montrul et al. (2011): "impossible," "probably impossible," "probably possible," "perfectly possible" (p. 44) or the scale used by Nabei and Swain (2002, p. 61): "absolutely correct," "probably correct," "probably incorrect," "absolutely incorrect." Some descriptions are more colorful, such as Schulz (2011)'s: "great," "okay," "strange," "awful," and "no intuition" (p. 327). Soler (2015, p. 634) gives descriptions along with numbers:

1. The sentence sounds really bad. You would never use it and you cannot imagine any NS using it.
2. The sentence sounds bad to you but not as bad as Example 1. You can imagine some NSs using this sentence.
3. You can't decide or the sentence doesn't sound too bad or too good.
4. The sentence sounds pretty good to you but not as good as Example 5.
5. The sentence sounds good to you. It's perfectly natural. You can imagine a NS using it.

TABLE 4.2 Sample scales and end point descriptors used in judgment task studies.

Akakura (2012)	1 (correct) to 4 (incorrect)
Bley-Vroman and Yoshinaga (2000)	−3 (completely impossible) to +3 (completely possible)
Cuza (2013)	−2 (odd) to +3 (fine) with intermediate values of slightly odd and more or less fine
Gabriele (2009)	1 ("I definitely cannot say this sentence in the context of this story") to 5 ("I definitely can say this sentence in the context of the story")
Montrul and Bowles (2009)	1 (completely unacceptable) to 5 (perfectly acceptable)
Prentza (2014)	−2 (ungrammatical) to +2 (grammatical)
Rothman and Iverson (2013)	1 (totally unnatural) to 5 (totally natural)
Soler (2015)	1 ("The sentence sounds really bad. You would never use it, and you cannot imagine any NS using it.") to 5 ("The sentence sounds good to you and you can imagine NSs using it")
Toth and Guijarro-Fuentes (2013)	1 (totally wrong) to 6 (excellent match)
Tremblay (2006)	−2 (sounds bad) to +2 (sounds good)
Zhang (2015)	−2 (completely/100% unacceptable) to +2 (completely/100% acceptable)

Others (e.g., Marsden, 2008 in a study of Japanese questions) use both numerical and written categories, as seen in Figure 4.1.

One important point to note about these scales is that they are not interval scales, as noted by Cowart (1997). That is, participants most likely do not interpret the difference between points as equal. For instance, participants may interpret the difference between *probably impossible* and *probably possible* to be greater than the difference between *probably possible* and *definitely possible* (see Ionin & Zyzik, 2014 for discussion). This fact may affect the analysis in that some statistics require an interval scale and, therefore, technically cannot be used with judgment data, an issue we return to in Chapter 6.

BOX 4.7 TYPES OF RATINGS AND SCALES EMPLOYED IN JUDGMENT TASKS

- Generally, a Likert scale will provide more information than a binary judgment, so in principle they are preferred. However, binary judgments may be preferable in conditions where a quick judgment is desired.
- It is often a good idea to include an *I don't know* or *I'm not sure* option, to try to eliminate guessing and make data interpretation clearer.
- To improve reliability, consider a Likert scale with 7 or 8 points, although 5 is common in SLA research. If a middle point is included, decide how you will label it and interpret it. In some cases, it may be preferable to use an even number of points to eliminate a hard-to-interpret middle point.
- Make sure your descriptors are clear for your participants. If you use a numeric scale, make sure you describe what the endpoints indicate.

4.2.8. Gradience of Judgments: Alternative Approaches

4.2.8.1. Using Lines

A few alternative approaches to traditional rating scales have been proposed. Two early studies using lines are White (1987), which investigated child learners (ages 11–12), and White (1989), which investigated adults and adolescents (age 15). In both studies, participants were required to mark on a line the degree of correctness of various sentences, with the center of the line equivalent to *not sure*.[2] The placement of a participant's line was equal to the perceived degree of correctness. For the analysis, a scale from .5 (*incorrect*) to 9 (*correct*) was imposed on the data.

4.2.8.2. Magnitude Estimation

Emphasizing the gradient nature of judgments is a methodology known as magnitude estimation. Though the methodology is used relatively rarely in L2 research, a handful of second language studies have employed it, or some variation of it. Even though magnitude estimation allows for fine-grained judgments in a manner similar to the White studies summarized in the previous section, there is a crucial difference: with White's use of a line, there is an upper and lower boundary for grammatical and ungrammatical, and the line length is fixed. In magnitude estimation, the scale is created by the participant and not imposed by the researcher.

Magnitude estimation has been demonstrated to give reliable results for sensory experiences such as length, brightness or loudness (Stevens, 1956, 1975). In this procedure, participants assign a number or other measurement (such as the length of a line) to the magnitude of a particular sensation in comparison to some norm. To give an example from the physical world, a participant might start out by rating the brightness of a lightbulb (the modulus). Participants may give the brightness of this bulb any numeric rating, such as "100," or draw a line to indicate the magnitude of the brightness. Then participants determine how much higher or lower a new lightbulb should be rated, based entirely on their own scale. If participants perceive the stimulus to be about twice as bright as the reference (the initial lightbulb), they may rate it as "200" or draw a line twice as long as the first, and if they perceive it as half as bright, they may rate it as "50" or draw a line about half as long. This approach can work for a variety of stimulus types, including pressure, loudness, length, and so on.

Some language researchers have argued that although linguistic judgments are more subjective than ratings of brightness or length, magnitude estimation can be effective at measuring grammaticality (Sorace, 1992, 2010, but see Featherston, 2008; Sprouse, 2011a; Weskott & Fanselow, 2011 for arguments against this idea). That is, data gathered by means of magnitude estimation correlate with results from Likert scales, rank ordering, and other typical methods of gathering judgment data (Bard et al., 1996; Cowart, 1997; Sorace, 1992). When magnitude estimation is used for judgments, the modulus is a sentence instead of a lightbulb or sound. Participants typically give it a rating with a number or by drawing a line and compare the acceptability of subsequent sentences to the modulus.

The advantage to using magnitude estimation is that the data can provide fine-grained distinctions in acceptability. For this reason, a number of L2 studies have used magnitude estimation to capture L2 judgments (e.g., Gass, Mackey, Alvarez-Torres, & Fernández-García, 1999; Kraš, 2011; Parodi & Tsimpli, 2005; Yuan, 1995). Hopp (2009) advocates for the use of magnitude estimation as a way of obtaining "maximally fine-grained judgments" (p. 470) when considering subtle differences based on discourse context. Magnitude estimation ratings can be analyzed with parametric statistics (they reflect interval data) once the ratings are converted into logarithms (see Chapter 6).

If magnitude estimation is used, there are several considerations regarding design. First, it is important to include stimuli with a wide range of grammaticality, including strongly grammatical and ungrammatical sentences, to ensure that data include clear points of reference for interpreting participants' responses. Second, a number of decisions must be made regarding the modulus, the baseline sentence to which other sentences will be compared. The first modulus may be given a fixed rating by the experimenter, or the participant may give it his/her own rating. The modulus may remain visible for comparison, or may be removed.

Instructions for judgment tasks with magnitude estimation are generally similar to those for judgment tasks using other types of rating scales. Sorace (2010, pp. 64–65) provides the following example:

INSTRUCTIONS FROM SORACE (2010, PP. 64–65)

The purpose of this exercise is to get you to judge the acceptability of some English sentences. You will see a series of sentences on the screen. These sentences are all different. Some will seem perfectly okay to you, but others will not. What we're after is not what you think of the meaning of the sentence, but what you think of the way it's constructed. Your task is to judge how good or bad each sentence is by assigning a number to it.

You can use any number that seems appropriate to you. For each sentence after the first, assign a number to show how good or bad that sentence is in proportion to the reference sentence.

For example, if the first sentence was:

1. cat the mat on sat the.

   and you gave it a 10, and if the next example:

2. the dog the bone ate.

   seemed ten times better, you could give it 100. If it seems half as good as the reference sentence, you could give it the number 5.

   You can use any range of positive numbers you like including, if necessary, fractions or decimals. You should not restrict your responses to, say, a 1–10 academic marking scale. However please do not use negative (minus) numbers or zero, because they are not proper multiples or fractions of positive numbers.

If you forget the reference sentence don't worry; if each of your judgments is in proportion to the first, you can judge the new sentence relative to any of them that you do remember.

There are no 'correct' answers, so whatever seems right to you is a valid response. Nor is there a 'correct' range of answers or a 'correct' place to start. Any convenient positive number will do for the reference.

We are interested in your first impressions, so don't spend too long thinking about your judgment.

Remember:

- Use any number you like for the first sentence.
- Judge each sentence in proportion to the reference sentence.
- Use any positive numbers you think appropriate.

BOX 4.8 USE OF MAGNITUDE ESTIMATION SCALES IN JUDGMENT RESEARCH

- When using magnitude estimation, as with other rating scales, make sure instructions are clear and give practice items.
- Make sure you have included some clearly grammatical and clearly ungrammatical sentences so that data can be analyzed accurately.

4.2.9. Confidence Ratings and Source Ratings

An increasing number of judgment task studies include confidence or source ratings. When they are included, confidence ratings are typically done after each rating of a target sentence in a judgment task. Participants indicate how confident they are in the rating that they gave for a particular sentence. Typically, the scale has four options (although more are possible): *guess*, *not confident*, *somewhat confident*, and *very confident*. Confidence ratings provide additional information about participants' knowledge of form and structure and help to mitigate the problem of random guessing by highlighting the extent to which learners resort to this strategy. Logically, a correlation between confidence and accuracy is expected, in that participants who are merely guessing may have more random or inaccurate responses. However, confidence ratings are sometimes used to try to discern the nature of participants' knowledge about grammaticality. An example can be seen in work by Grey, Williams, and Rebuschat (2014), who had participants press a "good" or "bad" button on a computer to respond to whether a given sentence sounded acceptable or not. Following each acceptability judgment, participants were asked how confident they were in their judgment. They were instructed to press 0 if they were *not confident*, 5 for *somewhat confident*, or 9 for *very confident*. The reasoning is that if participants perform above chance on the stimuli while claiming to merely be guessing at answers, they may have implicit knowledge about grammaticality of which they are unaware (see Rebuschat, 2013).

However, confidence ratings have their own shortcomings. One problem is that each participant decides subjectively the extent to which they are confident in their response, and individuals have varying criteria for what this means. Some people may report that they are guessing if they do not feel extremely confident in their rating, while others may report confidence despite having only slight intuitions about the sentence.

Source ratings may be asked for alongside confidence ratings. Here, participants are prompted to indicate what source of information their judgment was based on: for instance, whether they applied a grammatical rule or not. For example, Grey et al. (2014) used categories based on Dienes and Scott (2005) to ask about participants' reasons for their confidence ratings. They were asked to press *g* (for a complete guess), *i* (intuition), *m* (relied on memory of previous items), or *r* (used a rule in making a judgment). Typically, source ratings are used to try to determine whether participants possess implicit knowledge about the target grammar, or whether they are using learned or explicit rules to make judgments. Researchers may investigate whether accuracy scores correlate with various sources of knowledge. See Rebuschat (2013) for further discussion.

When asking for confidence and/or source ratings, the burden on the participant is increased in terms of cognitive load and time. If a researcher considers it important to understand confidence and/or source, the additional burden can be reduced in a number of ways. One possibility is to randomly select participants who respond to the confidence factor/source attribution. Another possibility, especially when there are numerous tokens of one target structure, is to request confidence/source ratings for a subset. A modification of these suggestions is to have some participants respond to some tokens and others to other tokens.

BOX 4.9 SOLICITATION OF CONFIDENCE AND SOURCE RATINGS

- Confidence and source ratings can be used to find out more about the nature of learners' knowledge.
- If it is burdensome to give confidence and/or source ratings to all sentences and if there are numerous exemplars of each sentence type, consider asking for ratings on a subset of sentences, rather than every single one.

4.2.10. Identifying and Correcting Errors

One of the main problems with traditional judgment tasks is that there is no way of knowing which aspect of a sentence a participant is responding to. For instance, a researcher may create the sentence *Every day I am getting up at 8:00 a.m.*, with the intention of examining whether learners understand the difference between simple and progressive aspect. However, a learner may decide that the preposition *at* should be *on*, and mark the sentence as ungrammatical for reasons having nothing to do with aspect. In fact, Kellerman (1987, p. 82) reports on a sentence written by a student: *But in that moment it was 6:00.* The teacher questioned the student and asked her about the preposition *in*. The student was convinced that the preposition was correct, but questioned whether the verb should be *had been* or *was*. In this case, the participant responded to a part of the sentence other than the one the researcher intended. Responses like these can damage the validity of the study. The damage is limited when stimuli are carefully controlled and an appropriate number of target items is included. However, to further guard against this problem, some judgment tasks prompt participants to indicate the problematic part of a sentence in their response. This can be done in a variety of ways.

Some researchers ask participants to underline, highlight, or circle the problematic part of a sentence if they mark it as ungrammatical. This approach helps eliminate responses where participants mark a sentence ungrammatical because of an irrelevant part of the sentence. This procedure is particularly simple when using binary scales (i.e., *acceptable/unacceptable*), because participants can be asked to add underlines only when they mark sentences unacceptable. However, it is also possible when using a scale with multiple points (e.g., *terrible, pretty bad, okay, good*). In these cases, participants are generally asked to indicate the problematic area of the sentence anytime they choose a response on the lower half of the scale.

There are some limitations to this method. Underlining, highlighting, or circling errors may not work for sentences where the problem cannot be easily limited to a portion of the sentence (e.g., *What do you believe the claim that Mary likes?*). Additionally, learners may extend the underlined part beyond the area with the error, leaving the researcher with the difficult task of interpreting where in the sentence the learner believed the error to be. Even in the best circumstances, underlining fails to provide information about what specific aspect of the underlined portion is found to be problematic. For this reason, some researchers ask participants to provide a reason why the underlined portion is incorrect. For instance, in a study investigating Spanish noun/adjective agreement, Leow (1996) asked participants to read each sentence, after which they were to select one of three possibilities (grammatically correct, grammatically incorrect, or not sure). This was followed by another set of instructions (p. 131):

1. If you select A (grammatically *correct*), please give a REASON(S) why you think it is correct.
2. If you select B (grammatically *incorrect*), please make the appropriate correction(s), and then give a REASON(S) why you made this correction.
3. If you select C (*not sure*), you don't need to give a REASON(S).

More commonly, however, researchers ask participants to provide a correction for sentences judged as ungrammatical, but do not ask for reasons when they mark the sentence correct.

Corrections can be provided in several different ways. Many researchers simply ask participants to cross out parts of the sentence they find unacceptable, draw arrows to move parts around, and write in new words where necessary. This may be easiest with paper-and-pencil tests, but making corrections is possible with judgment tasks presented on computers as well (e.g., White, Belikova, Hagstrom, Kupisch, & Özçelik, 2012). If sentences are short, it is possible to ask participants to rewrite the whole sentence correctly. In this case, some researchers may specify that only one change should be made, to discourage participants from making multiple changes (e.g., Coughlin & Tremblay, 2013). In other instances, responses that are unrelated to the structure being investigated (e.g., lexical choices, punctuation, pronominal use) are not included in the analysis (e.g., Cuza, 2013).

Corrections are perhaps the easiest to elicit when the test is written. However, it is possible to ask for corrections with an aural judgment task. For instance, Bianchi (2013) asked learners to repeat grammatical sentences and to change ungrammatical sentences to grammatical ones when they repeat them. This methodology is similar to an elicited imitation task (see Gass, 2018 for a review and the review and meta-analysis by Yan, Maeda, Lv, & Ginther, 2016).

Before administering a judgment task with corrections, researchers must decide how they will interpret possible responses. If a correction is made on the wrong part of the sentence, or if a participant underlines the wrong part of the sentence, the response is generally considered incorrect. If a correction is made to the right part of the sentence, but it is not fully correct, there are various ways to handle it. Sometimes partial scoring is appropriate. For example, Yalçin and Spada (2016, p. 249) examined the use of past progressive (e.g., *While they were eating in a café, the waiter dropped the dishes*). Participants received full credit (3 points) for correctly identifying ungrammatical sentences requiring past progressive (e.g., *My father slept when I left*) and for providing an accurate correction. If the correction was accurate in terms of aspect but not tense (e.g., *While they are eating in a café, the waiter dropped the dishes*), 2 points were given. If the correction left out the auxiliary (e.g., *She eating a sandwich at 9:00 last night*), only 1 point was given. Zero points were awarded if the correction did not change the ungrammatical verb form.

It should be noted that there may be disadvantages to having participants make corrections. One problem is that learners may accept sentences to avoid having to do the "extra" work of correcting them. Similarly, learners may sense that a sentence is incorrect but not be able to pinpoint the reason or supply a correction, and may therefore accept it. Another issue is brought up by Ellis (2004), who argues that judgment tasks that require learners to locate and/or correct answers may lead them to apply metalinguistic rules rather than using implicit knowledge to make judgments. One way to mitigate these problems was devised by Gass and Alvarez Torres (2005). In their study, they had participants make a binary judgment on sentences on a computer. When they were finished, all sentences that had been marked as "incorrect" were printed out and the participants made corrections at that point. This procedure had the advantage of allowing corrections so that the researchers knew if the targeted part of the sentence was being corrected without having to worry that the request for corrections affected judgments. Because corrections were done immediately upon completion of the task, the likelihood of memory issues was reduced. This methodology could also be used with auditorily presented judgment tasks, although we are not aware of any researchers who have employed this procedure.

BOX 4.10 INDICATING ERRORS IN SENTENCES

- If corrections are desired, give instructions carefully so that learners do not change or underline large portions of sentences, making responses difficult to interpret.
- Consider asking for corrections after judgments are made, to make sure that the ungrammatical part of the sentence is being appropriately targeted.
- Consider asking for judgments and corrections as two separate steps so that corrections will not affect judgments.

4.2.11. Modality

The most common means of presenting judgment tasks is in written mode. Part of the reason for the predominance of written judgment tasks is their convenience; that is, they can be created and presented relatively easily and can be reproduced for large groups if desired. Sentences may be presented on paper or computer screen. Additionally, it is possible to control the length of time that learners are exposed to written stimuli: written judgment tasks can be completely untimed, when participants can linger over material for as long as desired, or tightly controlled in an online setup (see Section 4.2.12).

Auditory judgment tasks are slightly more difficult to produce because an appropriate speaker needs to be found and good-quality recordings must be made. However, the decision of whether to use a written or audio judgment task goes beyond practicality. Murphy (1997) argues that audio judgment tasks are inherently more difficult than written judgment tasks. With a written task, participants can choose to read sentences at varying speeds or focus on various aspects of the input, but in audio judgment tasks, participants do not have control over the auditory signal, although this can be modified somewhat by allowing a participant to play a stimulus multiple times. Additionally, with audio judgment tasks, participants have to break the speech into words, while in written judgment tasks, the text is already broken up into words. A number of studies have shown that learners have lower accuracy on audio judgment tasks, presumably for these reasons (Haig, 1991;

Johnson, 1992; Murphy, 1997). Murphy (1997) also found that participants in an audio judgment task took longer to make judgments than did participants in a written judgment task, particularly on ungrammatical items, likely because making the judgments took more processing effort. Murphy points out that these issues may take on greater or lesser importance depending on the proficiency and learning context of a particular participant group; it is possible that highly advanced learners may perform equally well on both written and aural judgment tasks.

This issue raises another consideration regarding the modality of judgment tasks: participants' proficiency in specific skills. Listening skills will be a factor in an audio judgment task, while reading skills will be a factor in written judgment tasks. If learner groups are not matched for proficiency on these skills, or if their proficiency is too low, the validity of the task will be compromised. These effects could be magnified in cases where bound morphemes have particularly low acoustic salience or where a writing system is unfamiliar. Note, for example, the findings of Smith (2016), who found that native speakers of Japanese and English-speaking learners of Japanese failed to show grammaticality effects in a self-paced reading task, likely because of the participants' unfamiliarity with the adapted script that had been employed to make reading easier for the non-natives.

Some researchers propose that both written and audio stimuli should be presented simultaneously, which improves comprehension and recall of material (Frick, 1984). There are indeed some L2 studies that have taken this approach (see Parodi & Tsimpli, 2005; Bianchi, 2013 for examples), although it is less common. Murphy (1997) argues that limiting presentation mode to either reading or listening, without conducting the task in the other modality, limits researchers' understanding about learners' processing and knowledge. One study (Bialystok, 1997) presented half the sentences in a judgment task in written mode, the other half aurally.

For signed languages, judgment tasks can be presented with videos. See Cormier, Schembri, Vinson, and Orfanidou (2012) for an example.

BOX 4.11 MODALITY OF JUDGMENT TASKS

- Consider whether the visual or aural mode is practical for your purposes.
- Consider whether there will be difficulties for your participants in either listening or reading ability, and whether these factors will confound your results. Consider measuring learners' written or listening skills, especially when creating experimental groups.
- Remember that audio judgment tasks may be more difficult for some participants, although allowing multiple plays of a sentence mitigates this factor.
- Consider the related issue of timing (see Section 4.2.12).

4.2.12. Time Limits

A major concern with the design of a judgment task is whether or not there should be a time limit for responses. (See discussion in Chapter 2 regarding time limits as a way of distinguishing between implicit and explicit knowledge.)

For written judgment tasks, one possibility is simply not to have a time limit. This design was common throughout the early years of SLA research, partially due to the lack of widespread availability of computers. However, in recent years, untimed judgment tasks tend to be used with the understanding that they often elicit explicit knowledge. The issue of explicitness plays less of a role with some research, when the goal is to determine what knowledge learners have about a particular grammar issue. For instance, Hwang and Lardiere (2013) used judgment tasks to examine whether English-speaking learners of Korean knew the restrictions on the use of intrinsic *-tul*, a kind of plural marking. In this case, the researchers were not especially concerned about learners applying explicit knowledge because there is little instruction on *-tul* in language classrooms.

In other cases, studies using untimed judgment tasks are deliberately seeking to measure metalinguistic ability or explicit knowledge. Bowles (2011) examined the performance of heritage language learners on a variety of language tasks, including oral narration, oral imitation, a metalinguistic knowledge task, and timed and untimed judgment tasks. The author found that heritage language learners tended to perform the least well on tasks involving explicit knowledge, including the metalinguistic knowledge task and the untimed judgment task.

Researchers who want to encourage greater use of implicit knowledge by participants may choose to use a timed judgment task. There are a variety of ways to make a written judgment task timed. It is possible to time a pencil-and-paper task, with an overall time limit to complete all items. For example, Sabourin et al. (2006) provided participants with 30 minutes to complete 280 judgments. The downside of this approach is that it is impossible to control or measure how participants spend their time; for example, they could spend 25 minutes on the first half and then rush through the rest (or simply not finish). In principle, it is possible to regulate participants' attention to each item on a written judgment task by playing a tone every ten seconds or so and instructing them to move onto the next item, but this is rarely done.

The most common modern approach is to present written material on a computer. Using a computer to present a judgment task allows for tight control over the presentation of the material. The sentences can be made to appear on the screen for a precise amount of time; generally, the participant indicates a judgment by pressing a key, at which point the next sentence appears after a very slight delay. In this case, a decision must be made as to how long to allow the sentence to appear on the screen. There is no established amount of time that should be allowed. Many studies run an initial set of NS participants and then add an additional percentage to their reading times to allow for slower L2 processing. One possibility is to add 20% to native speaker median response times, as in Godfroid et al. (2015), Ellis (2005), and Loewen (2009). Another possibility is to use a predetermined amount of time, generally between six and nine seconds, depending on length and complexity of sentences (e.g., Della Putta, 2016; Gutiérrez, 2012). The time provided is generally longer if the judgment is made while the sentence is still on the screen (in which case the time for the judgment and the time for reading are combined) or if sentences are complex (see Section 4.3.2). Learners' proficiency must also be taken into account, so that sometimes longer time limits are provided. For example, Huang (2014) used 15-second time limits. Note, however, that if participants have long time limits, the task may begin to take on the quality of an untimed task. The goal is to allow enough time for processing the sentence fully but not enough time to think through the response multiple times, consider alternatives and learned rules, and so on. One way to avoid these issues is to simply ask participants to respond as quickly as they possibly can (e.g., de Graaff, 1997), but this is less common in recent research because of the lack of control over participants' exposure times. Piloting with comparable groups of participants can help researchers make appropriate decisions about time limits.

Timing an aural judgment task is a somewhat different matter. To a large extent, an aural judgment task is inherently timed because of the quick degradation of the speech signal. However, it is possible to reduce the time pressure in an aural judgment task by allowing the sentence to be played more than once, either automatically (e.g., Granena, 2014, in which each sentence in an aural judgment task was played twice) or under the control of the participants (e.g., Andringa & Curcic, 2015, in which participants could repeat sentences as often as they wanted).

In aural judgment tasks, a decision has to be made regarding how long to allow for the actual judgment after the presentation of each stimulus. If the participant fails to respond in the allotted time, the experiment typically moves to the next item. Three to four seconds per response, in addition to the time it takes to listen to the sentence, is common (e.g., Spada et al., 2015). The experiment may be designed to move on to the next item immediately once the participant responds, keeping the overall time of the experiment lower and encouraging quick responses. These response times can also be recorded for further information about participants' reactions to the stimuli. It is generally assumed that if participants take longer to respond to an item, they are responding to some aspect of the sentence that is ambiguous, complex, or anomalous in some way. Often ungrammatical sentences (that are recognized as such) take longer to respond to as participants struggle to process them.

BOX 4.12 TIMING JUDGMENT TASKS

- If there is concern about learners accessing explicit knowledge about the target form or structure, it is generally better to use a timed judgment task.

- Timing of paper-and-pencil judgments is difficult to control; generally, computers are used.
- Determine an appropriate time to allow a sentence to be viewed in a timed written judgment task, either by adding time to native speaker results or by using a formula established by previous research.
- If judgments are separated from sentence viewing or audio presentation, three to four seconds are allowed for a judgment before moving on automatically to the next item.
- With audio judgment tasks, it is common to allow the sentence to be played twice to ease the processing burden.
- Pilot the task before beginning the experiment to make sure the time limits are appropriate, the audio is clear, etc.

4.2.13. Participants

The choice of participants will obviously depend on the particular research question being asked. Participants need to be advanced enough to comprehend the sentences and to understand the instructions. Another concern is the participants' level of education. Acceptability judgment tasks, even those that are presented auditorily, may be problematic for participants who are unfamiliar with testing. In these cases, it may be necessary to carefully instruct participants in the methodology and provide multiple examples with feedback.

Although low levels of education can be a problem, it can be even worse to have learners with too much. In most studies, participants are excluded from recruitment or analysis if they are language specialists, such as students of linguistics or other language studies. Generally speaking, the concern with these learners is that they could be familiar with the methodology or the topic of interest; they may determine what the researcher is looking for and alter behavior accordingly. Students with a high level of study in a language are generally fine as long as the course of study does not involve courses in applied linguistics research (see discussion in Chapter 1 concerning expert and naïve judgers).

If groups are to be compared, it is important to ensure comparability of proficiency levels between or among groups. Care must be taken to ensure that detailed and appropriate proficiency data are collected. Bley-Vroman and Chaudron (1990) point out that groups that are being compared in productive tasks must be equated on production measures. This same notion can be applied to judgment data. If judgments are made on written data, measures that equate groups on their ability to read should be used; if an audio judgment task is being used, groups should be equated on their ability to comprehend the L2.

It is also generally wise to include a control group of participants who are native speakers of the target language and are similar demographically to the learner participants. The native speakers should perform very well on the acceptability judgment task; if they do not, problem items should be removed or the test should be redesigned.

Another factor that researchers need to determine is the number of participants for the study. It is possible to determine an appropriate number of participants by using a power analysis. This analysis determines the sample size that is needed to make a reasonable conclusion (see Sprouse & Almeida, 2017b for a discussion of power in experiments using acceptability judgments). Plonsky (2012, p. 201) defines power analysis as "a procedure designed to determine a priori the sample size necessary to reliably detect whether or not an effect will be found using inferential statistics." The following URL is a free calculator that can be used to calculate a minimal sample size based on whether a one-tailed or a two-tailed hypothesis is appropriate: www.danielsoper.com/statcalc/calculator.aspx?id=47 (retrieved 03/11/18).

Once you know how many participants you need, how do you find them? Sometimes finding enough participants can be challenging. Many researchers collect data in an online format (e.g., Qualtrics, Survey Monkey). This can be useful in allowing data to be collected at the researcher's own research site as well as asking colleagues elsewhere to distribute the data collection instrument to appropriate participants.

One new tool to aid in the search is Amazon's Mechanical Turk (referred to as MTurk), which is an online platform for collecting data. Its use for second language research is not widespread, but the possibilities are worthy of exploration particularly because MTurk's reach is international. Follmer, Sperling, and Suen (2017) point to advantages such as a diverse (age, geographical location) data pool and the facilitation of data collection with a large number of participants. Additionally, Sprouse (2011b) found that data collection took much less time with MTurk versus traditional lab experiments (in Sprouse's work, 88 hours over three months for traditional collection versus two hours for MTurk collection). Cost is another issue. All MTurk respondents are paid a minimal amount (Sprouse estimates a cost of $100 for 30 participants responding to 100 items). Importantly, Sprouse compared responses from MTurk and more traditional lab responses and found virtually no differences in the two contexts. A further elaboration of MTurk's value can be found in Enochson and Culbertson (2015), who investigated the use of MTurk with psycholinguistic measures such as response time. They found that it was possible to record precise timing measures using the platform.

However, there may be some disadvantages. Some have raised concerns about the reliability of data gathered through MTurk (see discussion in Mackey & Gass, 2016, pp. 40–43), partially due to the lack of information about participants, including their motivation for participating. Others argue against this point. For instance, Follmer et al. (2017) cite studies that compare MTurk data with other data and support the reliability of MTurk data.

At this point, there are not many studies that utilize crowdsourcing tools such as MTurk for second language data collection (cf. Evanini, Higgins, & Zechner, 2010; Negri & Mehdad, 2010; Kuperman, Stadthagen-Gonzalez, & Brysbaert, 2012). Given the difficulty and cost of recruiting participants, we anticipate that with careful investigation and scrutiny, crowdsourcing may be a way to increase sample size and hence the power of studies using judgment data. As an example, consider a study by Robenalt and Goldberg (2016) in which both native and non-native speakers of English were recruited by MTurk, resulting in a database of 157 native speakers and 276 English language learners. Thirty-nine different L1s were represented, although the bulk of them came from Hindi (33), Spanish (55), and Tamil (63).

BOX 4.13 PARTICIPANTS

- Consider running a power analysis to determine an appropriate number of participants for the study.
- Eliminate participants with knowledge of linguistics or applied linguistics.
- Keep in mind the level of education for participants. Participants with low levels of education may not be familiar with test-taking procedures and may process stimuli differently.
- Make sure any comparison groups have similar levels of education. (For instance, do not compare a group of low-literacy learners with a group of college-educated native speakers.)
- If you are comparing proficiency levels, use an appropriate proficiency measure. If using a written judgment task, use a written proficiency measure; if using an audio judgment task, use an audio proficiency measure.
- Consider using an online platform if recruiting participants in person is difficult.

4.2.14. Sentences in Context

There are many ways to conduct judgment tasks. It is frequently the case that sentences are presented in a decontextualized manner, one after the other with little semantic connection between them. This is particularly the case when a variety of language structures are being examined. However, in some studies, context is provided either through the use of videos or pictures or with additional text. Sometimes, these are provided simply to make the task more natural and to provide a more meaningful context. For instance, in Trahey's (1996) examination of adverb placement, experimental sentences were embedded in cartoon stories rather than simply listed one after the other (see Section 4.3.1 on using judgment tasks with children). Pictures can also be used to help participants better understand how a particular utterance could be interpreted. Providing a context might prevent a learner from rejecting a sentence simply because it is unusual or hard to imagine. For example, Bley-Vroman and Yoshinaga (2000) examined the acceptability of multiple *wh*-questions, such as *who is eating what?* (p. 10). While these questions could have been presented in isolation, pictures were provided to help learners visualize a possible context. For example, for the question *who is eating what?* a dog and pig are pictured, one eating carrots and one eating apples. Pictures are especially useful in helping learners imagine a possible context for similarly unusual sentences such as *who is singing where?* and *who is getting down how?* (p. 10).

More frequently, when additional context such as pictures or additional text is used, it is because context is necessary to ensure the proper interpretation of an utterance or to disambiguate between several possible meanings. For instance, Inagaki (2001) provided pictures to accompany sentences with motion verbs and goal prepositional phrases such as *Sam went into the house walking*, *Sam walked and went into the house*, or *Sam walked in the house for five minutes*. Pictures were necessary to ensure that participants interpreted the various sentences in the intended manner (i.e., something like *Sam walked into the house*) (p. 169). Juffs (2001) points out, though, that in some circumstances, videos might be necessary to ensure that participants make the intended interpretation. He gives the example of the Spanish sentence *El capitan marchó a los soldados* ("the captain marched the soldiers"), which might be accompanied by a picture of a captain standing next to soldiers, hastening them to march forward. However, the picture could feasibly be interpreted as "the captain marched *to* the soldiers" (p. 312). A video would make the difference clear. Indeed, videos have been used when a single picture would not suffice to ensure the intended interpretation. An example can be found in work by Nagano (2015), who used videos with sentences such as *the man vanished the coin* and *the coin vanished*, in order to make the role of agents and patients clear (p. 114).

A more frequent way that context is provided is with a sentence or story. Generally, this additional text precedes the sentence to be judged, and can be quite short. For instance, Cho (2017) examined the use of articles in English. She provided simple sentence pairs such as this one, where the learner had to make a judgment on the article in the second sentence (Cho, 2017, p. 376): *Jackie made a cake for the party. She served the cake with coffee and tea.* Where greater context is needed (for instance, with aspectual meanings), longer texts might be provided. An example comes from Gabriele (2009, p. 383), who examined tense and aspect using pictures with short stories such as the following: *Ken is an artist. At 12:00 he begins to paint a portrait of his family. At 8:00 he gives the portrait to his mother for her birthday.* The participants then had to judge a sentence with either a past tense verb, *Ken painted a portrait of his family*, or a present progressive verb, *Ken is painting a portrait of his family*.

In cases such as these, some researchers choose to not name the task *acceptability judgment* or *grammaticality judgment* but rather a name that highlights the fact that context is provided, such as *picture judgment task* (Montrul, 1999) or *story compatibility task* (Gabriele, 2009). Note that in these cases, all the sentences or utterances are grammatical. The task is to determine the fit between a particular utterance and a particular context.

In Chapter 5, we discuss these types of tasks in more detail.

BOX 4.14 PROVIDING CONTEXT

- In many cases, particularly when judgments are made on straightforward grammatical issues such as agreement marking, it is probably unnecessary to provide context.
- If context will help learners better understand how to interpret sentences, consider using text, picture, or video to provide it. Tasks involving fine semantic distinctions need to be very carefully designed to ensure that participants are interpreting sentences in the way the researcher intends.
- In all cases, pilot the task to make sure that the sentences are being interpreted the way you intend them to be.

4.3. Other Considerations

Thus far, in this chapter, we have focused on design features, presenting issues and controversies and making recommendations where appropriate. There are three final considerations that we raise: judgment tasks with children, complexity of stimuli, and proficiency.

4.3.1. Age

Most second language research that utilizes judgment data does so with adult or at least adolescent learners. Fallah, Jabbari, and Fazilatfar (2016) is an example of a study using judgment tasks with adolescents/older children. The participants were 13–14-year-old male Iranian students at the early stages of learning English (their L3). The task was a judgment task consisting of 40 test items (20 distractors and 20 target structures [possessive determiners and -*'s'*], ten of which were grammatical and ten of which were not). The pencil-and-paper task required that students indicate whether the sentence was "acceptable" or "unacceptable." The third possibility was an "I don't know" option. The results were used to test hypotheses regarding the dominant language with regard to the acquisition of a third language.

However, for young children, various adjustments are typically made to keep the attention of the participants, to improve the participants' understanding of the task, and to encourage the desired behavior. First, judgment tasks must be presented auditorily for very young children whose reading skills have not yet developed. It may be wise to use auditory judgment tasks up until age 12 or so, but certainly for children younger than 8. Second, more context is often provided in the form of pictures or video for children than for adults to make the task more natural. Frequently, puppets are used to interact with young children. For example, Barrios and Bernardo (2012), in a study with 7–8-year-olds, used a Mickey Mouse and Minnie Mouse puppet to provide experimental sentences with correct and incorrect case markings in Filipino, their second language. The puppets would "attempt" to describe pictures to the child using a friendly and clear voice. The child then said whether the puppet had described each picture correctly.

Using an even younger population, McDonald (2008), in a study with native-speaking children, used a judgment task with children as young as 6. Stimuli were presented aurally on a computer. After hearing each sentence, children were asked to push either the Z key (on which a smiley face sticker had been placed) for correct sentences, or the / key (on which a sad face sticker had been placed) for incorrect sentences. The target grammatical features included word order, yes/no questions, articles, *wh*-questions, plurals (regular and irregular), present progressive, past tense (regular and irregular), and third-person agreement. One hundred sentences (half grammatical and half ungrammatical) were included, and a break was given halfway through. For more discussion on creating judgment tasks for children, see McDaniel, McKee, and Cairns (1996).

4.3.2. Complexity

In Chapter 2, we dealt with the role that complexity might have when designing experiments that use judgment tasks as a way of measuring knowledge or learning. The topic has been dealt with in many ways. For example, Ellis (2004) brings in the construct of complexity as a variable when determining the amount of time to be allotted for each sentence. Cowan and Hatasa (1994) viewed the issue from the reverse perspective, pointing out the potential use of judgment data to determine complexity. In Chapter 2 (Section 2.6), we pointed to research where it is argued that acceptability judgments are, in part, determined by complexity (see Gibson & Thomas, 1999, for a similar finding). Hofmeister and colleagues, in a series of studies (e.g., Hofmeister, Culicover, & Winkler, 2015; Hofmeister et al., 2013; Hofmeister et al., 2012), consider issues of processing and complexity; however, we are unaware of L2 studies that directly explore the possibility that responses on judgment tasks may be influenced by difficulties involved in processing of complex sentences. Nonetheless, we raise this issue because it is likely to be an even more salient issue when dealing with non-native speakers than with native speakers.

4.3.3. Proficiency Level

Judgment data can be collected from virtually any level of proficiency. However, instructions should be tailored to the proficiency level of participants. Instructions for lower-proficiency participants should use simple, clear language and include plenty of examples. If the participants' proficiency is too low to easily understand the procedure, instructions should be given in the first language.

Careful descriptions of the participants' level are crucial. To categorize second language learners as beginning, intermediate, or advanced is meaningless without a specification of how those labels were determined. Standardized tests are ideal, but in many cases standardized tests are not available or would simply take too long; in such instances, it might be appropriate to use a tailor-made test to differentiate individuals. In other instances, the only possibility might be to describe the amount of language study. For English language study, describe the kind of program students are enrolled in. For instance, for university study, the participants could be in level three of a four-level prematriculation program; for study in the participants' home country, participants could be described as being in the last year of high school where English language study began in *x* grade. It is useful to describe the number of hours per week students had studies and the type of language exposure students have in and out of class. If information is available regarding the goals or standards of any program of study, this should also be included (e.g., by the end of fourth semester, students should have reached *x* proficiency level). Below we provide an example of a detailed description of participant proficiency levels.

BOX 4.15 DESCRIPTION OF PROFICIENCY LEVEL FROM GUTIÉRREZ (2013, PP. 430–431)

The participants were enrolled in one of two university-level courses of L2 Spanish and had returned a signed consent form. Twenty-nine of the participants were near the end of their third term of Spanish language instruction at the university; this level of instruction is intended to help learners develop their proficiency to a level similar to the A2 level of the Common European Framework of Reference (CEFR). The other 20 participants were close to completing their fifth term of Spanish language training; the goal is for learners to have reached a level similar to the B1 level of the CEFR at this point in their L2 development. All the participants were non-native speakers of Spanish. Twenty-two participants had taken Spanish language courses prior to university, most of them in high school. Forty-one participants started Spanish language training at the beginners' level at university, including 14 of the 22 who had taken Spanish previously but who did not meet the proficiency requirements of the intermediate level. The remaining eight participants had been placed in intermediate-level courses.

In other words, so that researchers can replicate results or do future analyses (e.g., meta-analyses), it is important to provide as much detailed information as possible.

4.4. Data Sharing

Issues of transparency have become important in scientific research, with the field of second language acquisition being no exception. The principle of reproducible research aims to provide scientific accountability by facilitating access for other researchers to the data upon which research conclusions are based. Following this principle, there is an open science movement that aims to make research procedures and data open and freely accessible. This includes making research articles accessible without cost and making actual data available to enable replication and determine reproducibility (cf. Gass, in press; Gass, Loewen, Plonsky, 2018 for more information). Reporting all aspects of research is essential to sound science so that others can understand and interpret what has been done in all aspects of a particular study. In the field of SLA, a digital repository of instruments for second language data collection, IRIS (www.iris-database.org), is a useful resource during study design. It is a free, searchable collection of materials and stimuli that have been used in published studies (cf. Marsden, Mackey, and Plonsky (2016 for further information). For example, it is possible to search the IRIS database for studies that have used judgments as a way of eliciting data.

4.5. Conclusion

This chapter has dealt with many design issues that need to be taken into consideration when planning a study using judgment data. Choices regarding length, timing, corrections, and more will have repercussions for participant behavior and results. Whatever choices are made regarding design, an important step is to pilot the study to work out potential issues before the experiment is run. Additionally, as the field moves toward greater transparency in research, it is crucial to provide detailed information about participants, procedure, and materials. These steps will allow future researchers to explore the findings of the study by either replicating it, expanding on it, or using the data from the study as part of a meta-analysis.

Notes

1. Based on the review of judgment data reported on in Plonsky et al. (in press), of the 385 judgment tasks reviewed approximately half (53%) used binary responses, with another 10% using binary responses in addition to an "I don't know" option.
2. White (personal communication, July 3, 2018) notes, however, that she now avoids the interpretation of the middle point of the line as *not sure*.

5

VARIATIONS ON JUDGMENT TASKS

5.1. Introduction

Acceptability judgment tasks can be defined as any tasks in which language users make decisions regarding the acceptability of particular utterances. This chapter deals with variations on judgment tasks by examining other types of tasks that serve the same function or a similar function to more traditional judgment tasks. We first deal with interpretation tasks (Section 5.2), which are similar to traditional acceptability judgment tasks; however, while traditional acceptability judgment tasks generally examine sentences that can be judged as grammatical or ungrammatical in isolation, interpretation tasks require participants to consider whether an utterance is appropriate in a particular situation. Similar to interpretation tasks are pragmatic judgment tasks (Section 5.3), in which participants judge whether an utterance is socially appropriate in a given context. We also deal with a few tasks that include aspects of judgment tasks but differ in the design. In Section 5.4 we discuss preference tasks, which require participants to determine which of two sentences is preferable, and in Section 5.5 we discuss error correction tasks, in which learners make changes to sentences to make them more acceptable. In Section 5.6, we introduce the possibility of using a multiple-choice format, and in Section 5.7 we discuss how psycholinguistic and neurolinguistic measures have been used with judgment tasks. Finally, we discuss tasks that incorporate several types of design (Section 5.8).

5.2. Interpretation Tasks

There are a variety of tasks that could be considered interpretation tasks, and a variety of designs with no established labels. Varied terms have been used, such as "picture matching task," "truth value judgment task," "context matching task," and so on. The key factor that unites these tasks is that participants must determine the appropriateness of a particular sentence or response within a particular context. In these tasks, the sentence or response to be evaluated is not ungrammatical per se, but it may or may not be natural or appropriate depending on the situation.

When the goal of the task is to rate the truth or accuracy of a statement in a context, the task is often referred to as a truth-value judgment task (TVJT). Typically, participants are first presented with a context, which is usually provided with a series of sentences or a paragraph, although pictures, videos, or even actors could serve the same function. Participants then judge whether sentences or utterances are appropriate given the context.

Reflexives are a frequent grammatical target in TVJTs (e.g., Eckman, 1994; Lakshmanan & Teranishi, 1994; Thomas, 1989, 1991, 1993, 1994, 1995; Wakabayashi, 1996; White, Bruhn-Garavito, Kawasaki, Pater, & Prévost, 1997). Reflexives have been an area of interest because speakers of different languages interpret the antecedent of a reflexive pronoun differently. For example, in Example 1 below is a sentence from Lakshmanan & Teranishi (1994, p. 187).

Example 1. John said that Bill saw himself in the mirror.

In this English sentence, "himself" refers to Bill and cannot be interpreted as referring to John. But this is not the case in all languages. The goal of this kind of research is to determine whether learners interpret "himself" as referring to John, Bill, or a third person. For example, in the Lakshmanan and Teranishi study, which examined the acquisition of Japanese by English-speaking learners, there was an English and a Japanese version of the task (p. 195):

Example 2. Japanese version

Sentence: Taroo-wa Jiroo-ga kagami-no naka-de zibun-o mita to itta (Taroo said that Jiroo saw himself in the mirror)
Response choices (one choice was to be circled):

a. zibun cannot be Taroo. agree disagree
b. zibun cannot be Jiroo. agree disagree

Example 3. English version

Sentence: John said that Bill saw himself in the mirror.
Response choices:

a. "Himself" cannot be John. agree disagree
b. "Himself" cannot be Bill. agree disagree

In a slight variation, Eckman (1994) used a picture identification task rather than just sentences. Participants saw two pictures and a sentence and had to indicate which picture the sentence described. They were told that the sentence could describe one picture, both pictures or neither picture. They were further told that before responding about one of the pictures, they should look at both pictures to see if both pictures were true reflections of the sentence.

A more elaborate context can also be introduced into truth value judgment tasks. For example, Ionin and Montrul (2009) examined article use by Spanish-speaking learners of English. They created short stories of 20–40 words with either specific or generic interpretations of a noun phrase. Each story was accompanied by a picture. The topic of one story was vegetarian tigers: "In our zoo, we have two very unusual tigers. Most tigers eat meat all the time. But our two tigers are vegetarian: They love to eat carrots, and they hate meat" (p. 159). Participants then rated one of the following sentences: *The tigers like carrots* (true); *tigers like meat* (true); or *these tigers like meat* (false). Note that in these cases, the goal of the tasks is not to examine correct or incorrect grammaticality per se. That is, the sentences would not be ungrammatical out of context. Rather, the tasks are examining the appropriateness of a sentence in a given context.

Another example comes from Glew (1998, p. 183). In this case, the response is indicated by a 'true/false' option.

Example 4. A boy and his father went on a bike ride together. The boy went down a hill very fast. "Don't go so fast!" shouted the father. It was too late; the boy fell off his bike and started crying. The father gave the boy a hug. Then the boy was happy again.

The boy was happy that the father hugged himself.
True False

As seen in these examples, there are many ways to design these tasks, with responses given as true/false judgments, picture selections, and so on. Contexts must also be carefully designed. Generally, the goal of providing context is to disambiguate possible interpretations. This can be tricky at times. For instance, in Glew (1998, p. 179), one question (shown in Example 5) had to be removed from analysis because it led to ambiguous interpretations.

Example 5. Context: Teresa and Madeleine went to a party one night. Teresa drank too much beer at the party. When it was time to go home, Teresa was worried because she didn't want to drive her car. "I'll drive you home," said Madeleine. "Oh, thank you Madeleine. I really appreciate it," said Teresa.

Teresa was happy that Madeleine drove herself home.
True False

The planned response was "false," but the researcher was surprised to find that many participants had responded "true." It became apparent that this was technically possible; while it is strongly implied that Madeleine drove Teresa home, it is certainly possible that Madeleine drove (herself) home afterwards, as well. Thus, the item turned out to be ambiguous and the response may have reflected that ambiguity rather interpretation of the referent of the reflexive pronoun.

Tasks requiring participants to determine how well language fits a particular context may be given other names, such as "context matching" or "picture matching," avoiding the use of the term "judgment" entirely. For example, in a study by McManus and Marsden (2017) of English-speaking learners of French, the researchers used what they referred to as a "context matching task" to measure treatment effects. The task consisted of a context in English and a French stimulus sentence that either matched or did not match the meaning expressed in the English context. The target of investigation was the French imperfect and in particular the difference between a habitual or ongoing function of the imperfect. Examples 6 and 7 are examples of a matched (acceptable) and a mismatched (unacceptable) condition respectively (McManus & Marsden, 2017, p. 470):

Example 6. Matched trial

Context (ongoing):

> Yesterday, Patrick was expecting his wife to come back from work any minute. Just as he was on his way out, she appeared in the driveway.

Stimulus (ongoing):

> Quand Patrick quittait la maison, il a vu sa femme. (When Patrick was leaving the house, he saw his wife.)

Example 7. Mismatched trial

Context (ongoing):

> Yesterday, Patrick was expecting his wife to come back from work any minute. Just as he was on his way out, she appeared in the driveway.

Stimulus (habitual):

> Quand Patrick quittait la maison, il voyait sa femme. (When Patrick left the house, he used to see his wife.)

The task was done on a computer and the context remained on the screen for ten seconds. This was followed by the French stimulus, which was presented orally for the listening task and in writing for the writing task. Participants were to determine how good the match was between the meaning of the context and the stimulus by pressing a number on the keyboard. The choice was from 1 (very good) to 5 (very poor) with an additional option for "I don't know." See Ionin (2012) and Ionin and Zyzik (2014) for further discussion on interpretation tasks such as those described in this section.

5.3. Pragmatic Tasks

Judgment tasks are most frequently used to examine learners' ability to evaluate grammatical appropriateness, but they have also been used to investigate pragmatics. In these types of judgment tasks, participants are generally asked to rate the appropriateness or naturalness of responses to a particular context, in terms of politeness, friendliness, or some other social factor. For example, Li (2012) examined requests in L2 Chinese by speakers of a variety of first languages. The author used a task called a "pragmatic listening judgment task" to evaluate how well learners understood pragmatic norms in Chinese after instruction. Participants heard a context in English and then a request made in Chinese. They then had to determine whether the request was appropriate or not, as in Example 8 (Li, 2012, p. 413).

Example 8. Context: Yesterday, Professor Wang gave out some handouts in the class. Ma Yang didn't come to the class due to illness. Ma Yang wants to get a copy of the handout from Professor Wang. Ma Yang explains situation and says 王老师，您能不能给我一份讲义？ (Professor Wang, can you give me a copy of the handout?)

a. pragmatically appropriate and grammatically accurate
b. pragmatically inappropriate and grammatically accurate
c. pragmatically appropriate and grammatically inaccurate

Similarly, Bardovi-Harlig and Dörnyei (1998) investigated pragmatic and grammatical judgments. They created 22 videos with scenarios including requests, apologies, refusals, and suggestions. In the videos, several actors portrayed a social situation that ended with a particular response. Participants viewed the videos twice; the second time, after the final response the scene froze for seven seconds to give participants time to mark an answer sheet that included the targeted response (see Example 9 below). Some utterances were grammatically correct but pragmatically inappropriate; some were grammatically incorrect but pragmatically appropriate; and some were both grammatically and pragmatically well-formed. An example is given in Example 9. (Bardovi-Harlig & Dörnyei, 1998, p. 241).

Example 9. Context: I'm really sorry but I was in such a rush this morning and I didn't brought it today!

Was the last part appropriate correct? ☐ Yes ☐ No

If there was a problem, how bad do you think it was?

Not bad at all ___:___:___:___:___:___Very bad

Results indicated that English language students and teachers studying in their home countries ranked grammatical errors to be worse than pragmatic errors, while ESL students and teachers in the United States considered pragmatic errors to be more serious.

In a study examining use of and beliefs about stigmatized language forms, Zaykovskaya (in progress) used a judgment task for both native and non-native speakers of English. Her object of investigation was the use of English remarkable "like,"[1] for example, "there are *like* twenty students in that class." Zaykovskaya devised a judgment task, referred to as a "syntactic perception task," in which participants heard a sentence played on a laptop. The sentences were taken from a large corpus of native speaker speech. Instructions asked participants to indicate how natural the sentence sounded to them. To provide a response, participants chose a number ranging from 1 (unnatural) to 5 (perfectly natural). Interestingly, preliminary results indicate that native speakers rated sentences using 'like' as unnatural, despite the fact that the sentences were taken from native speaker speech. It is likely that the native speakers rejected the sentences because they consider "like" to be a marker of uneducated speech. These results indicate that using judgment-type tasks for certain pragmatic targets may be problematic. (See Chapter 1, Section 1.2.4.)

5.4. Preference Tasks

In a preference task, participants are typically presented with two sentences and asked which they prefer. Preference tasks thus differ from traditional acceptability judgments in that participants are not required to determine whether utterances are acceptable or not. Instead, they indicate which choice seems better. This means that even if participants find all sentences to be acceptable or unacceptable, they still make a choice for one over the other. This format may be particularly suitable in cases where researchers want to compare specific options that are hypothesized to exist in participants' grammar. For example, researchers may want to compare a structure that is allowed in the target language versus one that is allowed in the first language, or a target structure versus a hypothesized default option.

Particularly in earlier research, many tasks labeled "preference tasks" were a hybrid between a preference task and a judgment task, in which participants made judgments of each sentence. The main difference between this design and other judgment tasks was that the sentences were deliberately contrasted with each other. For instance, in a study of frequency and manner adverb placement, where the concern was the effects of positive and negative evidence, White (1991) used two written tests as measures of effectiveness: a judgment task and what she called a preference task, but which, in actuality, might be better thought of as a comparison task, terminology she uses in her 1989 paper where the same methodology was used. Her participants were French-speaking learners of English in grades 5 and 6. Participants were presented with two sentences with five options, as in Example 10:

Example 10. Sentences from White (1991)'s preference task (p. 142):

1. Susan often plays the piano.
2. Susan plays often the piano.

Response choices:

a. only 1 is right
b. only 2 is right
c. both right
d. both wrong
e. don't know

White argued that this design had the advantage of limiting "what the subject has to think about, since two sentences are presented for consideration which differ only in syntactic form" (p. 142).[2] That is, the task functions as a judgment task in which attention is directly focused on the particular issue of interest, in this case, adverb placement before or after the verb.

A similar design was used in a 1999 study by Spada and Lightbown. French-speaking ESL students in the sixth grade (ages 11–12) participated in a classroom intervention study investigating English question formation. Of the four tasks used to determine knowledge of questions, one was a preference task. Pairs of sentences were presented to participants, and, as in the White (1991) study, learners had to determine which ones were correct or indicate that they didn't know. The study also included distractors. Example 11 presents two pairs of sentences from their study.

Example 11. Sentences from Spada and Lightbown (1999, p. 9).

A. The teachers like to cook?
B. Do the teachers like to cook?

A. Can I take the dog outside?
B. Do I can take the dog outside?

In all cases, the following response options were given for each pair:

a. only A is correct
b. only B is correct
c. A and B are correct
d. A and B are incorrect
e. don't know

The authors compared the results of the preference task with an oral production task and suggested that recognition of correctly structured questions was more accurate than production.

These types of preference tasks can also include context to make interpretation of the target sentences clearer. For example, Geeslin and Guijarro-Fuentes (2006), in their study of Portuguese speakers learning Spanish as an L2, used a "contextualized preference task." The context was provided by a paragraph that was related to the preceding paragraph. In other words, a story was created (see discussion below regarding the 2008 study by the same authors). Participants could accept one of two options or both, but they could not reject both. The focus was the use of the verbs *ser* and *estar* in Spanish, which both translate to the verb 'be' in English. The researchers provided context and then two sentences, one with *ser* and one with *estar*. Instructions were as follows:

> Pretend you are attending a university in a Spanish-speaking country. You will read descriptions below of situations that have taken place between your friends Paula and Raúl. They live together, but they are not romantically involved. Read each sentence and decide which of Raúl's responses you prefer. Please check only one option.
>
> *(p. 103)*

Example 12 is an example of the context and the options (Geeslin & Guijarro-Fuentes, 2006, p. 103).

Example 12. Context: Paula and Raúl leave the apartment and go to a local restaurant. They eat there frequently and the people who work there are always very nice. This time, Raúl has ordered something new on the menu and Paula is curious about what Raúl thinks of the food.

Question: Paula: Raúl, do you like your food?
Possible answers to be evaluated by participant:

A. "Yes, dinner is good" (*ser*)
B. "Yes, dinner is good" (*estar*)

Response choices (one choice was to be circled by the participant)

a. I prefer sentence A
b. I prefer sentence B
c. I like both A and B.

Another example of a task that is a hybrid of a preference task and a judgment task is Guijarro-Fuentes and Larrañaga (2011). In this study of the acquisition of verbal morphology and verb movement by English learners of Spanish, there were four tasks, one of which was a traditional judgment task (using a 5-point scale) and another a "preference judgment task," in which learners indicated a preference for one of a pair of sentences, and then indicated whether the sentence that they rejected was grammatical or not. An example is given in Example 13 (p. 519).

Example 13. Sentences to be evaluated:

1. Pedro corre regularmente tres millas. (Pedro runs regularly three miles.)
2. Pedro corre tres millas regularmente. (Pedro runs three miles regularly.)

This preference task had clear similarities with a traditional judgment task.

Preference tasks can also be designed without asking participants to make judgments. With this design, preference tasks are particularly well-suited to situations in which there is no clear grammatical or ungrammatical option, when traditional sentence-level judgments may provide data that are difficult to interpret. For instance, Valenzuela et al. (2012) examined code-mixed Spanish/English language in what they referred to as a "sentence selection task." They asked two groups to respond to sentences that followed a conversation. One group was comprised of heritage speakers (simultaneous bilinguals) and the other of L1 Spanish/L2 English speakers. The researchers combined Spanish determiners with English nouns to examine whether speakers preferred determiners that agreed in gender with the Spanish translation of the English noun, or if they preferred masculine determiners, which are typically a default. Each sentence was preceded by a dialogue. Participants had to state which of the sentences was more natural. There were two types of sentences: sentences with a determiner phrase (DP), and sentences with copulas and adjective agreement. Examples are given in 14–17 (Valenzuela et al., 2012, p. 488).

Example 14. Code-switched DP (feminine)[3]

Dialogue: Juan: I had lots of fun anoche [last night], pues [then], I ran into Sergio.
Elisa: Seriously? ¿Dónde lo viste? [Where did you see him?]

a. En la (f) party [at the]
b. En el (m) party [at the]

Example 15. Code-switched DP (masculine)

Dialogue: Juan: ¡Qué despiste! [How forgetful!] I totally forgot something.
Elisa: ¿Que te olvidaste? [What did you forget?]

a. La (f) wine
b. El (m) wine

Example 16. Agreement/copulas (feminine)

Dialogue: Elisa: Ayer fue el cumpleaños de Fernando. [Yesterday was Fernando's birthday.]
Juan: Really? And how was the party?

a. Fue fantástica (f) [it was fantastic]
b. Fue fantástico (m) [it was fantastic]

Example 17. Agreement/copulas (masculine)

Dialogue: Juan: ¿Qué hay de beber? [What do you have to drink?]
Elisa: All I have is BC wine.

a. Fine, es exquisita (f) [that's great]
b. Fine, es exquisito (m) [that's great]

In this case, neither option can be said to be grammatical or ungrammatical, making a preference task a good choice.

Some researchers argue that preference tasks are also particularly suited to cases where differences in acceptability are subtle and difficult to articulate. For instance, Stringer, Burghardt, Seo, and Wang (2011) investigated spatial modifiers in English with 121 learners from 17 L1 backgrounds. Participants heard two sentences and then indicated which they thought was more acceptable. For example, participants heard *He flies straight on over the camels* and then *He flies on straight over the camels*. They then indicated whether they preferred the first sentence or the second. The researchers argued that this format, more than a traditional judgment task, could capture initial reactions to the stimuli. In particular, they were trying to make it possible to give a quick response and not consider alternate pronunciations that changed stress and intonation. Finally, perhaps most important, they wanted to prevent participants from indicating that they had no intuitions due to the somewhat indeterminate nature of this particular task.

Like judgment tasks, preference tasks can also include pictures or text that provide context for an interpretation. For example, Cuza and Frank (2015) investigated double complementizer questions in Spanish. They provided a short text to introduce a context and then asked participants to indicate which sentence most logically followed it. For example, "Sandra told John how much she paid for the car, and John asked her: To whom did you pay so much money?" The participants had to choose how to say "John told Sandra who she paid so much money." They could choose either *Juan le dijo a Sandra a quién le pagó tanto dinero* [John told Sandra who she paid so much money], or *Juan le dijo a Sandra que a quién le pagó tanto dinero* [John asked Sandra who she paid so much money] (Cuza & Frank, 2015, p. 15).

Geeslin and Guijarro-Fuentes (2008) provided a more elaborate context in their study examining the choice of copula in Spanish (*ser* vs. *estar*) by English speakers. Their context consisted of a paragraph that included discourse and sentence-level variables that typically predict which Spanish copula to use. Particularly innovative was the use of a continued narrative: the 28 "contexts" were embedded in a long story. In Example 18, we give an example of the opening context (two examples), the middle (two examples), and the end of the story (two examples).

Example 18. Sentences from Geeslin and Guijarro-Fuentes (2008).
The participants were to indicate whether the form of the verb *estar* or *ser* was the better option or if both could be used.

a. Context (beginning examples):

1. Paula and Raúl are planning to go out to dinner. Paula is yelling from the bedroom while she gets ready in order to make plans with Raúl. As she comes out of her room she asks:

   Paula: Do you want to go in my car?
   Raúl: ¡Ay! ¡Qué bonita estás/eres! [How pretty you are!]

2. Paula says thank you and asks if their friend Pablo will be joining them for dinner. Paula wants to talk to him about their math class. Raúl says that Pablo isn't coming and Paula wants to know why:

   Paula: Why isn't Pablo coming?
   Raúl: Porque no le llamé antes y ahora está/es enojado. [Because I didn't call him and now he is mad.]

b. Context (middle two examples)

1. Paula and Raúl have been having trouble coordinating their schedules. Since only Paula has a car, Raúl has to know which days he has to take the bus. During the day, Paula has come up with a suggestion that will save him some bus fare:

   Paula: You can come with me in the morning and go with Juan in the afternoon.
   Raúl: ¡Ay! ¡Qué inteligente estás/eres! [How intelligent you are!]

2. Even though Raúl likes Paula's idea she realizes there might be a problem. Sometimes Juan has trouble with the police because he drives too fast. Raúl says he doesn't mind that but he does mind Juan's way of dressing. Paula is curious about what he means:

   Paula: Why don't you like his way of dressing?
   Raúl: ¡Esta semana su pelo es/está azul! [This week his hair is blue!]

c. Context (final two examples)

1. Paula tells Raúl that his reaction surprises her. She didn't realize he had already met Alicia. Raúl starts to laugh at Paula because Paula has not realized that Alicia and Raúl are from the same hometown. Paula doesn't understand:

   Paula: Why are you laughing?
   Raúl: ¡Nunca eres/estás despierta! [You are never aware of things!]

2. Paula and Raúl arrive at the apartment again. Paula comments that she ate a lot and she will have to eat less tomorrow.

   Paula: I ate so much that I am going to start to gain weight.
   Raúl: Pero Paula, tú estás/eres muy delgada. [But Paula, you are so thin.]

By allowing a choice between the two verbs, the possibility of the participants focusing on unrelated aspects of the sentence is reduced.

As the above examples have demonstrated, preference tasks involve a forced choice; that is, participants must indicate a preference for one or the other. However, some researchers allow for a third "I don't know" option, similar to what is sometimes made available in judgment tasks, to prevent participants from guessing if they do not have a particular preference.

Not surprisingly, preference tasks require many of the same design choices that judgment tasks do. They can be auditory or written; they can be timed or untimed; they can have fillers, and so on (see Chapter 4). Additionally, similar issues about implicit and explicit knowledge arise with preference tasks; that is, timed or auditory preference tasks may be more likely to elicit decisions based on implicit knowledge than untimed written ones, although this is not fully established in research (see Chapter 2). Many researchers who use preference tasks also conduct traditional judgment tasks and compare the results (e.g., Guijarro-Fuentes & Larrañaga, 2011). Typically, the results point to a similar conclusion, as is the case in Stringer et al. (2011).

5.5. Error Correction Tasks

As we noted in Chapter 4, some judgment tasks require participants to not only judge whether sentences are acceptable or not, but also to indicate the location of the unacceptability or to correct it. In this section, we deal with error correction tasks that include the second part without the first; that is, participants are asked to find and correct errors but not to make judgments on sentences directly. For instance, in White and Ranta's (2002) study of the use of *his* and *her* by French-speaking learners of English, the authors used what they called a passage correction task. Learners read a story and identified and corrected a number of possessive determiner errors, along with errors in various distractors. The researchers argued that this task does not "require 'metalingual' knowledge but does require that the learner have an analyzed representation of the grammatical rule" (p. 274). Similarly, Hu (2002), in a study of the acquisition of six English structures by Chinese learners of English, used a timed and untimed error correction task in addition to a spontaneous writing task. In the error correction tasks, learners of English were presented with 60 sentences with errors and asked to correct and rewrite them. Examples of the sentences are given in Examples 19–23 (Hu, 2002, p. 385).

Example 19. A woman and an old man came to see John. Old man introduced himself as John's uncle.
Example 20. Cow is a useful animal.
Example 21. When he came back from his holiday, he brought three things: old watch, beautiful knife, and new camera.
Example 22. Foreign correspondent is a reporter who is stationed in a foreign country by a news agency.
Example 23. There are the beautiful flowers and apple trees in my garden, where I work and spend my spare time.

One of the issues with tasks such as these is that learners may correct perceived errors that are actually grammatically correct. For instance, Hu (2002) found that the learners often rewrote sentences fairly extensively, changing both the target structure and a number of other, grammatical, structures. To avoid this issue, some researchers provide direction in locating errors. For instance, Zhang's (2012) error correction task included 20 sentences with four segments underlined in each. The participants' task was to first identify which part of the sentence contained an error, and then to correct that part (and that part only). In scoring the task, Zhang awarded one point for a correct identification of the location of the error and one point for an appropriate correction.

Some error correction tasks leave out identification of the error altogether and ask for a correction only. For instance, Rodríguez Silva and Roehr-Brackin (2016) provided sentences with highlighted portions. Participants had to correct the error in that portion and provide a grammar rule to explain it (see Ziętek & Roehr, 2011, for a similar task). On the other hand, tasks can be created in which learners locate errors from a selection of possibilities. These are often framed as multiple-choice tasks (see Bauer, 1991 for an example).

Error correction tasks may be timed or untimed. (See Hu's study from 2002 for an example of a study using both timed and untimed error correction tasks.) While it is possible that timed error correction tasks may encourage the use of implicit knowledge more than untimed error correction tasks, these tasks are generally not viewed as a good measure of implicit knowledge (Ellis, 2005); even a short amount of time to complete the task might give participants time to access explicit knowledge.

5.6. Multiple-Choice Tasks

In some cases, researchers show participants a sentence and then provide choices from which a participant can select one or more responses. The task may be set up similarly to a cloze task. For example, Birdsong and Flege (2001) investigated regular and irregular morphology in English. Participants were native speakers of Spanish and Korean. As shown in Example 24 below, they had to determine the appropriate way to inflect nouns and verbs by choosing from five possible responses (Birdsong & Flege, 2001, n.p.):

Example 24. 1. Low Frequency Regular Noun Plural

There are five ________ on each hand.

a. knuckli
b. knuckle
c. knuckles
d. knackle
e. knuckleses

2. High Frequency Irregular Verb Past

Yesterday the little girl ________ for the first time.

a. swim
b. swam
c. swimmed
d. swims
e. swammed

The researchers considered both response time and accuracy in their analysis.

5.7. Judgment Tasks in Combination With Psycholinguistic and Neurolinguistic Measures

Judgment tasks have been used in combination with various psycholinguistic and neurolinguistic measures, such as self-paced reading, eye-tracking, Event Related brain Potentials (ERPs), functional magnetic resonance imaging (fMRIs), and so on. In these cases, the judgment task often serves two purposes: first, it gives participants a task that encourages them to read sentences carefully while various measurements are taken, and second, it provides accuracy and reaction time data that help in the analysis of results.

For instance, Juffs and Harrington (1996) investigated the processing of English embedded finite and nonfinite clauses by speakers of Chinese and a native speaker control group. The participants read 114 sentences encompassing 20 syntactic structures, including grammatical *wh*-questions with long distance *wh*-movement (see Example 25) and ungrammatical *wh*-extractions (see Example 26) (p. 296). Word-by-word reading times were examined for both the native speakers and the non-native speakers.

Example 25. *Who$_i$ does Bill believe t$_i$ to hate the manager?
Example 26. *What$_i$ did Sam see the man who stole t$_i$?

Also included were a variety of "garden path" sentences that encouraged readers to take a certain interpretation and then change it, as in Example 27 (p. 297).

Example 27. ?After Bill drank the water proved to be poisoned.

In these cases, the judgment data were particularly important. If a participant rated the sentence as grammatical, it was expected that increased reading times would be seen as the reanalysis is taking place (i.e., realizing that *drank* is intransitive rather than transitive in this context). However, if the participant rated a sentence as ungrammatical, it was expected that reading times would not be as elevated because no reanalysis had taken place. Indeed, it was found that both native and non-native speakers judged many grammatical garden path sentences to be ungrammatical, and that in these cases the pattern of reading time per word was different than when the judgment was made correctly. Judgment response times (that is, the time it took to make a judgment) were also analyzed, with longer times interpreted as indicating difficulty with parsing.

Overall, the researchers concluded that Chinese-speaking ESL learners differed from native speakers in their parsing of a number of grammatical phenomena in English, and that these parsing issues may account for certain differences in performance that had previously been attributed to a grammatical deficit. The methodology used in this task has been used for other experiments, often labeled an "online self-paced grammaticality judgment task." See Perpiñan (2015) for an example.

Similar to self-paced reading studies are those using eye-tracking. For example, Tuninetti, Warren, and Tokowicz (2015) examined the effects of cue strength and first language influence on sensitivity to ungrammaticalities in a second language. Arabic- and Mandarin-speaking learners of English read sentences and provided binary acceptability judgments while their eye movements were tracked. Two types of ungrammaticalities were included, as shown in Examples 29 and 30. Example 28 is the grammatical version (Tuninetti et al., 2015, p. 569).

Example 28. She pulled the short skirt up over her leggings.
Example 29. *She pulled skirt the short up over her leggings.
Example 30. *She pulled the skirt short up over her leggings.

Accuracy percentages on judgments for each sentence type were compared between the Arabic-speaking group, the Mandarin-speaking group, and a native speaker control group. Additionally, a variety of measures were examined from the eye-tracking data, including first fixation duration, regressions out of the target area, first pass reading times, go-past time, and total reading time. The researchers did not find strong evidence for first language transfer effects and argued that the extremely salient nature of the ungrammaticalities in this study (i.e., changes in article and adjective word order) probably overrode the possibility of observing transfer effects. They noted that the participants, including native speakers, performed more accurately on ungrammatical than grammatical sentences, which is fairly unusual.

In a study using Event Related brain Potential recordings, Weber-Fox and Neville (1996) investigated language processing in Chinese–English bilinguals who had their first exposure to English at different ages. Specifically, they recorded ERPs while participants read sentences such as the following examples and made a judgment regarding whether the sentences were "good English sentences" or not (p. 233).

Example 31. Semantic/pragmatic control and violation:

a. The scientist criticized Max's proof of the theorem.
b. *The scientist criticized Max's event of the theorem.

Example 32. Phrase structure control and violation:

a. The scientist criticized a proof of the theorem.
b. *The scientist criticized Max's of proof the theorem.

Example 33. Specificity constraint controls and violation:

a. The scientist criticized Max's proof of the theorem.
b. What did the scientist criticize a proof of?
c. *What did the scientist criticize Max's proof of?

Example 34. Subjacency constraint control and violation:

a. Was the proof of the theorem criticized by the scientist?
b. *What was a proof of criticized by the scientist?

Both judgment accuracy and ERP recordings were examined. Judgment accuracy was lower in the groups that had been exposed to English at a later age.

Additionally, this group showed the largest differences from the native speakers in their ERP results. The authors concluded that their findings demonstrated support for a critical or sensitive period for language learning.

More recently, Morgan-Short and her colleagues have similarly gathered neuroimaging data from participants as they make judgments. For example, Faretta-Stutenberg and Morgan-Short (2018) collected EEG data from participants as they made judgments on L2 Spanish sentences in addition to assessments of both declarative and procedural learning abilities and measures of working memory capacity. Some participants were on their home university campuses and others were at a campus in an L2 environment. Using these varied measures of individual differences, they were able to determine the predictive value of cognitive abilities on processing and linguistic knowledge as a function of learning setting (see also Faretta-Stutenberg & Morgan-Short, in press for a study using a similar methodology, in this case considering imaging and behavioral data as well as data related to differences in cognitive abilities to understand differences in levels of proficiency and amount of contact in a study-abroad context).

Grey, Sanz, Morgan-Short, and Ullman (2018) also used ERP data collected while participants were judging the grammaticality of sentences. That study focused on differences between monolinguals and bilinguals in the learning of a new (artificial) learning. Their participants did not show differences in the behavioral measures used, one of which was a judgment task. A combination of these data types allowed the researchers to suggest that even when there are no behavioral differences, bilinguals are more like native speakers.

5.8. Many Task Types in One

A recent entry into the scene comes from Hartshorne, Tenenbaum, and Pinker (in press), who used the internet to collect data from 669,398 native and non-native speakers of English. Data were analyzed through a computational model with the goal of determining language learning ability, taking into account age (current), age of first exposure, and years of experience with the language. The researchers supported the idea of a critical period after which language learning becomes more difficult, but with a later starting point than many have argued for.

Data were collected through an internet site (http://archive.gameswithwords.org/WhichEnglish/). Instructions were given online as follows: "In this quiz, you will decide which sentences are grammatical (correct) and which are not" (n.p.). Interestingly, a variety of judgment task types were used (Hartshorne et al., in press). For example, one task was to read the sentence "The dog was chased by the cat" and match that sentence with one of two pictures (a picture of a dog chasing a cat and another of a cat chasing a dog) (see Section 5.2 on interpretation tasks). In another example, the sentence "Every hiker climbed a hill" was presented with instructions to click on the picture that best matches the sentence. The two pictures are presented in Figure 5.1:

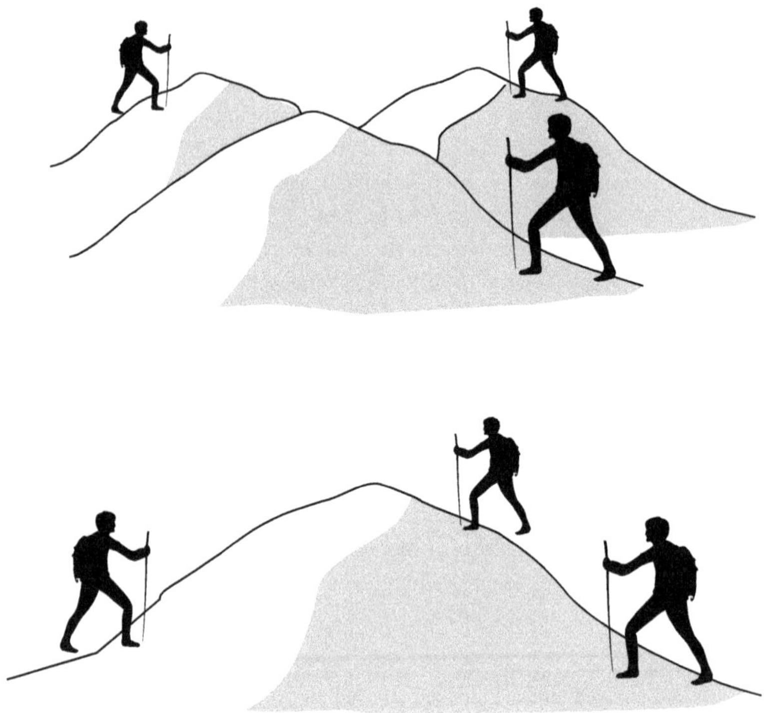

FIGURE 5.1 Every hiker climbed a hill

Source: From "A critical period for second language acquisition: Evidence from 2/3 million English speakers" by J. Hartshorne, J. Tenenbaum, & S. Pinker, in press, *Cognition*, by Elsevier. Reprinted by permission (picture is from survey on which article is based).

In other cases, the prompt is: which of the following sentences sounds natural? Possible responses are given in Example 35. Here, the design is similar to the studies by White (1991) and Spada and Lightbown (1999).

Example 35. a. I shan't be coming to the party after all.
b. I won't be coming to the party after all.
c. Both
d Neither

In another case, respondents were told to: "Fill in the blank. Check **all** correct answers" (n.p.). For example, see Example 36.

Example 36. The people ________ angry.

a. is
b. be
c. were
d. are

In another task, a list of unrelated sentences was presented, as in Example 37 below, with instructions to check all sentences which were grammatical.

Example 37. Response Choices

a. John agreed the contract.
b. Sally appealed against the decision.
c. I'll write my brother.
d. I'm just after telling you.
e. The government was unable to agree on the budget.
f. I after ate dinner.
g. Who did Sue ask why Sam was waiting?
h. He thought he could win the game.

In sum, in this innovative study of the critical period hypothesis, the researchers drew upon a range of tasks (Hartshorne et al., in press) discussed in this chapter.

5.9. Conclusion

Many tasks that researchers ask participants to perform require some evaluation of nativelike and non-nativelike language. While we have included a variety of tasks in this chapter, including context matching tasks, pragmatic judgment tasks, preference tasks, and error correction tasks, we have not attempted to describe every task that is related to judgment tasks. In the next chapter, we focus on the analysis of judgment tasks and how judgment data are handled.

Notes

1. Zaykovskaya gives the following five examples of this use of *like* in English, taken from D'Arcy (2017).

   1. **Quotative complementizer**: And we were like, "Yeah but you get to sleep like three-quarters of your life." He WAS LIKE, "That's an upside." (2/f/12)
   2. **Approximative adverb**: It could have taken you all day to go LIKE thirty miles. (N/f/76)

3. **Discourse marker**: Nobody said a word. LIKE my first experience with death was this Italian family. (N/f/82)
4. **Discourse particle**: Well you just cut out LIKE a girl figure and a boy figure and then you'd cut out LIKE a dress or a skirt or a coat, and like you'd color it. (N/f/75)
5. **Sentence adverb** (largely restricted to certain dialects of English spoken mainly in Ireland, Northern Ireland, northeast of England, and Scotland): You'd hit the mud on the bottom LIKE. (TEA/62m/1941)

2. White's judgment task sentences were given in the context of a story, although the story itself did not affect the meaning. Only the form (adverb placement) was of concern.
3. Masculine and feminine in these examples refers to the gender of the noun in Spanish. We have only provided examples for nouns that end in -o or -a. Other nouns (e.g., those ending in -e or in consonants) were also included in the study.

6

ANALYZING JUDGMENT DATA

6.1. Introduction

In earlier chapters, we dealt with the use of judgment data in linguistic and second language research. In Chapter 4, we elaborated on many of the important considerations that must be dealt with when designing a study in which judgment data are used. In Chapter 5, we considered alternatives to traditional judgment tasks. In this chapter, we focus on what happens after data have been collected. In particular, the focus is on the analysis of judgment data.

6.2. Cleaning the Data

Before doing any statistical analyses or even presenting raw data, it is necessary to make sure that there are no inaccurate, corrupt, or incomplete data points. This is often referred to as cleaning the data.

6.2.1. Stimuli

As has been mentioned elsewhere in this book, pilot testing is a crucial step before data collection actually takes place. Unfortunately, it is possible that potential problems are not revealed in this initial phase. Therefore, one of the first steps when looking at data is to check the responses on the judgment task (based on pilot data or actual data if the experiment has already been conducted) to make sure that there are no items that may have been confusing or misleading in ways that are irrelevant to the issues of interest. One way to determine which items may be problematic is to see which grammatical items have unexpectedly low accuracy scores and which ungrammatical items have unexpectedly high scores from native speakers or another control group. These items should be edited and re-checked by additional pilot testing (if the experiment has not yet been run) or removed (if the experiment has already been run). Unfortunately, there is no definitive threshold at which it becomes clear that a particular item is problematic. This is particularly true given that studies vary widely on the nature of the grammatical phenomena being investigated. Most researchers simply "eyeball" the results and determine whether any one item or group of items stands out as performing differently than the others. In other words, this is a judgment call and should be reported when writing up results.

For example, in Spinner (2013), one goal was to determine whether participants were sensitive to adverb placement. One of the sentences that was expected to be less acceptable to native speakers was *John heard yesterday the song on the radio* (as opposed to *John heard the song on the radio yesterday*). However, native speakers rated the sentence higher than expected. Debriefing interviews with participants who had participated revealed that some had interpreted the sentence as "John heard the song 'Yesterday' (by the Beatles) on the radio" (p. 74). Therefore, the sentence could not be included in its original form. To minimize the number of items that need to be modified, it is advisable to run the judgment task with a control group. After running the judgment task, examine the accuracy scores for unexpected results and conduct interviews with participants in which they have a chance to look over the items and report on which were problematic for them. This procedure will make it possible to adjust problematic items before administering the experiment. Keep in mind, however, that even in the best of worlds, pilot testing does not resolve all problems (see Mackey & Gass, 2016, pp. 52–53 for a discussion of the role of pilot testing).

Another example is reported by Tremblay (2005), who discovered a problem with an item after running the experiment, so that it was too late to edit the item.

> an important typo was found in one of the tokens, which led half the participants to reject the sentence when it was meant to be grammatical. To maintain the number of tokens appearing in each condition equal, the score on this item was replaced by the participant's mean on that sentence type.[1]
>
> *(p. 137)*

Note that it is not only unexpectedly low or high accuracy on an item that may indicate its problematic nature. If a large number of participants skip an item entirely or rate it "I don't know," this may also indicate that it needs to be edited or removed.

6.2.2. Participants

Schütze and Sprouse (2013) make the important point of eliminating outliers. In particular, "the pre-processing of numerical judgment data . . . is common to all data in experimental psychology: the identification of participants who did not perform the task correctly, and the identification of extreme outliers in the responses" (pp. 42–43). They also point out that "there are as yet no generally agreed upon procedures for participant and outlier removal for acceptability judgments" (p. 43).

In order to check whether participants seemed to be paying attention during the task, and whether they understood the instructions, researchers may eliminate participants who do not score above a certain level on certain items, such as fillers. Typically, participants who score lower than 70% or 80% on these control items are eliminated from the analysis. The assumption or justification in doing so is that they are not able to complete the task appropriately, either because they are not focused, have proficiency that is too low, or for any other reason. An illustration of elimination, albeit in a sentence-matching task, comes from Duffield, Matsuo, and Roberts (2007), who make this explicit whey they state:

> One participant correctly matched the experimental items only 48% of the time; this was 2 standard deviations below the mean of the group (94.7%), and therefore this participant's data were removed from subsequent analyses, since it was not clear that she had paid attention during the experiment.
>
> *(p. 168)*

Researchers may use different accuracy scores on filler items to eliminate participants, depending on the research interest. For example, Oh (2010) used a 50% accuracy criterion on ten filler items; Marsden (2008), on the other hand, eliminated participants if they had more than one inappropriate answer to the ten distractor items (90% accuracy). Another possibility is to include a few key screening sentences to eliminate anyone who does not rate all of them as expected. For instance, Robenalt and Goldberg (2016) had three practice trials with one unambiguously acceptable sentence and one unambiguously unacceptable sentence. Participants who did not rate these unambiguous sentences as expected were eliminated from analysis, on the grounds that they probably did not understand the task or were not paying attention.

It may also be a good idea to eliminate participants who rate a high proportion of sentences "I don't know," who skip a large number of sentences, or who seem biased to inappropriately respond "no" or "yes" to a high proportion of fillers. The number of participants that are eliminated from analysis for any reason should be reported along with the reasons for elimination. As noted above, there is no clear cutoff point of accuracy or bias for participants who should be eliminated. For better or worse, determining which participants to cut tends to be more art than science, but in general, a good rule of thumb is to eliminate individuals who seem to be responding to the task differently than the rest of the group. Generally speaking, only a small proportion of participants will be removed from analysis. If a researcher needs to eliminate more than 5–10% of participants because of performance issues on the judgment task, there is possibly a problem with the study design (including the appropriateness of the task in relation to the proficiency level of the participants), with the instructions, and/or with the stimuli themselves.

6.2.3. Reliability

Another way to evaluate whether the judgment task is measuring what it is designed to measure is to investigate the internal consistency of the task. The purpose of measuring internal consistency is to ensure that the items in the test generally correlate with each other, indicating that the test items reliably measure the same construct or constructs. This check has become common practice, with Cronbach's alpha (α) being the measure that is most often used. It is generally agreed that a score of above .70 is acceptable for reliability (see Larson-Hall, 2016), although higher numbers are preferable as they indicate that the dataset contains less 'noise' or measurement error. However, observed estimates of reliability in L2 research are actually often somewhat higher. Looking across 1,323 instruments used in published L2 research, Plonsky and Derrick (2016) found a median estimate of internal consistency of .82, and Plonsky et al. (in press) found a median reliability coefficient of .8 (interquartile range = .15). If the value of Cronbach's alpha is outside the interquartile range, the amount of error in the data may put into question any subsequent findings. If this is the case, problematic items may be removed after data collection. Ideally, of course, it is preferable to check reliability before collecting experimental data; for this reason, once again, pilot testing is important, and this step should not be skipped or compromised. An example of a reliability table for judgment data comes from Zhang (2015, p. 473), where reliability is presented for four tests, an elicited imitation task, a timed judgment task, an untimed judgment task, and a metalinguistic knowledge test. Zhang also separated out the grammatical and ungrammatical items from the timed and untimed judgment tasks.

TABLE 6.1 Reliability values of the tests (N = 100)

Test	*Reliability Coefficient*
Elicited Imitation Test	α = .76
Timed GJT (TGJT)	α = .70
Untimed GJT (UGJT)	α = .72
Metalinguistic Knowledge Test	α = .76
TGJT—Grammatical Items	α = .83
TGJT—Ungrammatical Items	α = .63
UGJT—Grammatical Items	α = .70
UGJT—Ungrammatical Items	α = .72

Source: From "Measuring university-level L2 learners' implicit and explicit linguistic knowledge" by R. Zhang, 2015, *Studies in Second Language Acquisition*, *37*, p. 473. Published by Cambridge University Press. Reprinted by permission.

BOX 6.1 CLEANING THE DATA

- Pilot your judgment task with participants from your target population(s) to ensure that your materials are working as intended and measuring what you intend to measure.
- Eliminate or replace items that native speakers do not respond to as expected.
- Evaluate the reliability of your task with Cronbach's alpha. It should be over .70, preferably higher. If it is not, edit your task.
- For items that did not perform well during your experiment, it is generally best to remove the item from analysis.
- Consider including some performance checks in your judgment task, for instance, items that are clearly grammatical or ungrammatical. If your participants do not generally respond to these items as expected, they may be confused or not paying attention; eliminate those participants from analysis.
- Report in detail how you edited your judgment task, eliminated participants, and checked reliability.

6.3. Scoring Responses to Binary and Scalar Judgments

6.3.1. Binary Judgments

Typically, binary judgments are scored rather simply, by assigning 1 point to correct responses and 0 to incorrect responses. This is the case for both grammatical and ungrammatical items. Percentage accuracy is then calculated by adding up the points and dividing by the total number of items. For instance, if a learner judged 7 out of 10 items correct, her accuracy score is .7 or 70%. Typically, if an item is left unanswered, it is considered an incorrect (or 0) response. Similarly, if a participant responds with an "I don't know" option, these items are typically scored as incorrect, under the assumption that the participant lacks the intuition or ability to make a judgment. This corresponds to indeterminate sentences described in Chapter 2, which refer to those sentences about which a learner has no intuition. In other words, 'I don't know' options (whether overtly stated or implied by a lack of response) suggest minimally that those sentences are not part of the internal grammar of the learner, where grammatical knowledge includes knowing what is grammatical and knowing what is ungrammatical. For example, Gutiérrez (2013, p. 433) counted responses left unanswered as incorrect. His rationale is as follows:

> GJTs were scored in terms of correct versus incorrect answers. Although items left blank could be interpreted as (a) the participants not being sure

> about the grammaticality of the sentence or (b) the participants not having had enough time to judge the sentence, a decision was made to count such an answer as incorrect for purposes of comparability with [other studies].

Another option is to remove these responses from analysis, with the assumption that the participant may not have understood the item or may have been confused by it in some unknown way.

Many studies using binary judgments combine participants' responses on grammatical and ungrammatical items for analysis, giving one overall mean score. However, there are several important reasons to analyze them separately. Ellis (2005), following research from Bialystok (1979) and Hedgcock (1993), reported that grammatical and ungrammatical items can function differently in judgment tests. Specifically, in Ellis' study ungrammatical items correlated more strongly with explicit, metalinguistic measures, while grammatical items correlated more strongly with implicit measures (see Chapter 3, Section 3.3.1, for a discussion of this issue). Because of these findings, some researchers choose to focus on responses to either grammatical or ungrammatical items. For example, Spinner (2013) analyzed responses to grammatical items on a timed judgment task in an effort to tap into implicit knowledge of L2 participants, while Erlam and Loewen (2010) examined ungrammatical items in an effort to measure explicit knowledge. For most purposes, however, it is recommended to present accuracy on both grammatical and ungrammatical items separately. In fact, in some cases, participants are found to respond quite differently to them. For instance, Andringa and Curcic (2015) examined participants who were presented with an explicit rule (explicit learners) and those who were not (implicit learners). They found that both groups scored highly on grammatical items, but the implicit learners scored significantly less accurately on the ungrammatical ones. The authors reason that the implicit learners had a strong preference for judging sentences to be grammatical. This important finding would not have been available if the analysis had combined the results for grammatical and ungrammatical sentences.

6.3.2. Scalar Responses

If a Likert scale is used, percentage accuracy is not calculated. Instead, Likert scale results are often analyzed by assigning a number to each point on the scale (e.g., "terrible" = 0, "quite bad" = 1, "pretty good" = 2, "perfect" = 3) and taking mean results for grammatical and ungrammatical items separately. Researchers who use Likert scales with a middle point (i.e., an odd-numbered scale) may consider the middle point to be the equivalent of "I don't know" or "unsure." In this case, the middle point is typically averaged into the results as usual; however, this type of analysis is not ideal because it cannot distinguish between lack of knowledge (see Chapters 3 and 4) and a judgment of a neutral point between acceptable and unacceptable. To avoid this problem, many studies include an "I don't know" option along with the Likert scale but separate from it; as noted above, these responses are then typically removed from analysis altogether (see Toth, 2008 for an example), although they could also be reported separately, for instance by determining which items garnered the most "I don't know" choices.

As another way to examine scalar data, accuracy scores can be calculated by collapsing a scale into correct and incorrect responses. For example, in a four-point scale from 1 (unacceptable) to 4 (acceptable), scores of 3 and 4 might be considered accurate responses to acceptable stimuli, while scores of 1 and 2 are considered inaccurate. Akakura (2012) asked participants to judge sentences on a scale that included correct, probably correct, probably incorrect, and incorrect. For the analysis, she used only correct and incorrect; in other words, she changed scalar data into dichotomous data.

> Participants were given unlimited time to judge 20 underlined portions of sentences for grammaticality, both grammatical (n = 10) and ungrammatical (n = 10) . . . . A confidence assessment measure was incorporated within the judgement scale with the coding: 1. correct, 2. probably correct, 3. probably incorrect and 4. incorrect, forcing participants to make a judgement. If the sentence was grammatical, correct answers included both 'correct' and 'probably correct'. Responses were scored as either correct (1 point) or incorrect (0 points).
>
> *(p. 19)*

The results from collapsing a scale could be presented along with average ratings to provide information that mean scores can obscure. This presentation may be particularly useful when learners respond inconsistently to some of the tokens of a grammatical structure, for instance marking some as acceptable and some as unacceptable. In these cases, mean scores may make it appear that learners find sentences to be about halfway between acceptable and unacceptable, when in reality they have mixed judgments.

BOX 6.2 SCORING JUDGMENT DATA

- Create an accuracy score for ungrammatical and grammatical items. Report these scores separately.
- Assign a numerical score to Likert scale judgment and report average scores for native and non-native speaking participants.
- Generally, "I don't know" responses or lack of response is considered an inaccurate response.

- Decide what to do with the middle point of a scale, if there is one. It can be averaged in with other scores, keeping in mind that the middle point is ambiguous as it can mean 'I don't know' or it can be a true 'middle-of-the-road' response.
- Consider reporting "I don't know" responses (if they are included) separately.

6.4. Scoring Corrections

In Chapter 4, we discussed the role of corrections. When corrections are requested, decisions must be made on how to score them. If participants mark a grammatical item "good" and make no correction, or if they mark an ungrammatical item "bad" and make the appropriate correction, the item is easy to score. However, there are times when participants do not behave in these predictable ways. For instance, participants may mark a grammatical item as bad but then make a correction to an irrelevant part of the sentence. For instance, in a study investigating subject–verb agreement, a participant may mark the sentence *My favorite food is pizza* bad, but erroneously change the word "favorite" to "best." In this case, it is reasonable to ignore the correction and classify this response as correct because subject–verb agreement, the target, is correct. Similarly, a participant may mark an ungrammatical item as bad but make the wrong change. For instance, in the same study, if the participant changed *My favorite food are pizza* to *My best food are pizza,* it is reasonable to classify this as an incorrect response because the erroneous target (subject-verb agreement) is not detected as an error. Some responses may be on the right track but not quite target-like, which can make them difficult to classify. For example, if the sentence is *My favorite food are pizza* and the participant changes it to *My favorite food was pizza,* the participant indicated the location of the problem but unnecessarily changed the tense. In these cases, one option is to use partial scoring (for instance, ½ point instead of a full point) because the learner knew the correct item to change and fixed the agreement error, but did so in a way that was not complete and accurate. Giving partial credit for choosing the right area of the sentence to change is reasonable as it can indicate that knowledge is developing (see, e.g., Gass, Svetics, & Lemelin, 2003; Gass, 1983). Yalçin and Spada (2016, p. 249) describe their procedure for partial scoring as follows.

> Partial scoring was also used for the passive GJT. When learners accurately corrected an ungrammatical passive sentence (i.e., a sentence missing either the auxiliary 'be', or the past participle '-ed'), they received two points. If they failed to provide the past participle form of the main verb, while correcting an ungrammatical sentence, they were given one point (e.g., "The

> tires on the car were change"). The provision of "be" auxiliary and the past participle form of the main verb were required components to obtain full points. Minor spelling errors for past participle forms were ignored as long as there was an attempt to provide the form.

However, not every researcher makes this choice. Falk and Bardel (2011), for example, required participants to both mark a sentence as bad and also to make an accurate correction for a response to an ungrammatical item to be scored as correct. In their study, items were labeled "hits" or "misses." A response was a "miss": "1) if the participant judged a grammatical sentence as ungrammatical and either made an incorrect correction or no correction, or 2) if the participant judged an ungrammatical sentence as grammatical" (p. 70). Any decision will depend to some extent on the nature of the ungrammaticality (for instance, whether it is even possible to make a partial correction, as might be the case with complex syntax) and on the type of knowledge that the researcher is trying to measure.

Sometimes very fine-grained decisions on corrections must be made. For example, Izumi, Bigelow, Fujiwara, and Fearnow (1999, p. 426) used judgment data to investigate second language learners' performance on past counterfactual structures (e.g., *If Ann had traveled to Spain in '92, she would have seen the Olympics*). In their task, participants circled the ungrammatical part of the sentence. However, some learners circled portions of the sentence that were larger than they needed to be, thereby including other parts of the sentence as well. The authors considered the response to be accurate if the circle included up to two words before or after the location of the error (to some extent, an arbitrary choice). Their analysis is detailed below (pp. 433–434).

Decision 1

Is there a circle whenever a no response was chosen? If the answer is 'no,' the sentence was excluded from the analysis.

Decision 2

Is the conditional-related part circled? If the answer is 'no,' the sentence was excluded from analysis. If the answer was 'yes,' another decision was needed.

Decision 3

Is there a correct judgment of grammaticality? Here there were four possibilities:

1. If the response was 'yes'
    a. The sentence was correct = 1 point
    b. The sentence was incorrect = 0 points

2. If the response was 'no'
    a. The sentence was correct = 0 points
    b. The sentence was incorrect: another decision was needed.

Decision 4

Is the appropriate clause identified (circled)?

a. No = 0 points
b. Yes = 1 point

Decisions about how to score corrections should be made before the experiment begins. Pilot testing will help determine problem areas so that they can be resolved early.

BOX 6.3 SCORING CORRECTIONS

- Make decisions about how corrections will be scored before beginning the experiment. In particular, decide what to do if a participant corrects ungrammaticalities in an ambiguous way. We recommend only including those instances that are unambiguous. Alternatively, if ambiguous responses are included, it should be made clear in the final write-up in what way they were ambiguous and what decision was made about inclusion.
- Generally, full points are awarded if participants make no corrections to grammatical sentences, or if they correct an unrelated part of the sentence.
- Generally, full points are awarded if a participant corrects the appropriate part of an ungrammatical sentence.
- Consider giving partial credit if a participant only partially corrects ungrammaticalities.

6.5. Basic Inferential Statistics With Judgment Data

6.5.1. Descriptive Statistics

Most studies with judgment data compare responses between groups or between conditions (or both). Typically, where binary judgments are collected, an average accuracy score is taken for each group and/or each condition, often separating grammatical and ungrammatical items. These means, along with standard deviations, are presented, often in graphic or tabular form, as in the example from Zhang (2015, p. 473). In his study, there were four tests, an elicited imitation test, two judgment tests (timed and untimed), and a metalinguistic knowledge test. In Table 6.2 are the descriptive statistics for the four tests as well as the descriptive statistics of the two judgment tasks divided by grammatical and ungrammatical sentences.

Where scalar judgments are collected, mean ratings for groups and/or conditions are presented. An example of a table of descriptive statistics with scalar data comes from Tremblay (2005, p. 149), in which she investigates native speaker intuitions of factive items (*John knew what Mary was doing* and **John knew what was Mary doing*) and questions (*Did Bill wonder where Keith is going shopping* and **Did Bill wonder where is Keith going shopping*). In this study, participants rated sentences from 1 (ungrammatical) to 4 (grammatical). See Table 6.3 for a display of her data.

TABLE 6.2 Descriptive statistics of the tests (N = 100)

Tests	*Items*	*M*	*SD*
EIT	34	.44	.12
TGJT	68	.51	.10
UGJT	68	.86	.08
MKT	40	.56	.12
TGJT G	34	.69	.18
TGJT UG	34	.33	.12
UGJT G	34	.85	.10
UGJT UG	34	.87	.10

Note. EIT = elicited imitation test; TGJT = timed grammaticality judgment test; TGJT G = timed grammaticality judgment test grammatical items; TGJT UG = timed grammaticality judgment test ungrammatical items; UGJT = untimed grammaticality judgment test; UGJT G = untimed grammaticality judgment test grammatical items; UGJT UG = untimed grammaticality judgment test ungrammatical items; MKT = metalinguistic knowledge test.

Source: From "Measuring university-level L2 learners' implicit and explicit linguistic knowledge" by R. Zhang, 2015, *Studies in Second Language Acquisition*, *37*, p. 473, by Cambridge University Press. Reprinted by permission.

TABLE 6.3 Means and standard deviations for grammatical and ungrammatical control, experimental, factive, and question items

Sentence Type	*Mean*	*St. Dev.*
Grammatical		
Control	3.90	.22
Experimental	3.58	.41
Factive	3.86	.20
Question	3.76	.27
Ungrammatical		
Control	1.13	.19
Experimental	1.76	.40
Factive	2.43	.61
Question	2.37	.43

Source: From "Theoretical and methodological perspectives on the use of grammaticality judgment tasks in linguistic theory" by A. Tremblay, 2005, *Second Language Studies*, 24, p. 149. Reprinted by permission of A. Tremblay and J.D. Brown.

6.5.2. Comparisons Between Groups: t-Tests and ANOVAs

After examining descriptive statistics for general patterns, more formal comparisons between groups or conditions can be made with *t*-tests or ANOVAs. One example comes from Roberts and Liszka (2013), who elicited acceptability ratings (scale = 1–6) on English tense/aspect agreement violations. To compare group performance, a Type (match, mismatch, i.e., acceptable/unacceptable) by Group (English NS, French L2 learners, German L2 learners) ANOVA was conducted on both past simple and present perfect items. Post-hoc comparisons with a Tukey HSD adjustment were conducted for all significant effects and interactions. The researchers first presented Tables 6.4 and 6.5 (p. 423). This is followed by a verbal description of the statistical analyses.

> the analysis, which found a main effect of Type (F1 $(1, 57) = 61.17$; $p < 0.001$; $\eta^2 = .52$; F2 $(1, 23) = 44.27$; $p < 0.001$; $\eta^2 = .66$), and a main effect of Group (F1 $(2, 57) = 4.14$; $p < 0.05$; $\eta^2 = .13$; F2 $(2, 46) = 15.68$; $p < 0.01$; $\eta^2 = .66$). However, post-hoc Tukey HSD test found no significant differences between the groups (ps > .07).
>
> *(p. 423)*

TABLE 6.4 Acceptability judgments: past simple (SD is given in parentheses)

	Match	*Mismatch*
English native speakers	4.27 (1.0)	3.24 (1.3)
French L2 learners	5.10 (0.7)	3.49 (1.2)
German L2 learners	4.98 (0.9)	3.82 (1.2)

Source: From "Processing tense/aspect agreement violations on-line in the second language: A self-paced reading study with French and German L2 learners of English" by L. Roberts & S. Liszka, 2013, *Second Language Research*, 29, p. 423. Sage Journals. Reprinted by permission.

TABLE 6.5 Acceptability judgments: present perfect (SD is given in parentheses)

	Match	*Mismatch*
English native speakers	4.57 (1.1)	2.53 (1.5)
French L2 learners	4.80 (0.8)	3.08 (1.3)
German L2 learners	4.79 (0.9)	3.90 (1.2)

Source: From "Processing tense/aspect agreement violations on-line in the second language: A self-paced reading study with French and German L2 learners of English" by L. Roberts & S. Liszka, 2013, *Second Language Research*, 29, p. 423. Published by Sage Journals. Reprinted by permission.

As can be seen, the authors also report the post-hoc comparison, in this case, Tukey HSD. This is important because when multiple comparisons are made with ANOVAs and the F value is significant, one needs to pinpoint the location of the differences with a post-hoc comparison such as Tukey, Scheffé, a Bonferroni correction, or a Duncan's multiple range test.

Most commonly, these comparisons between groups and conditions are made with a 'by-participants' analysis, because in most studies the assumption is that the participants are sampled as representatives of the population under investigation. However, it is also the case that the items are taken to be representatives of some phenomenon under investigation; therefore, a 'by-items' analysis is also appropriate (see Cowart, 1997). The by-items analysis provides information about the consistency of the responses for individual items in the judgment task. For example, if some of the sentences within a particular condition are responded to differently than others, the by-items analysis may not be significant even if the by-participants analysis is. From a psycholinguistic perspective, a predictor should only be considered significant if both the by-participants and by-items analyses show a significant effect (Baayen, 2008; Forster & Dickinson, 1976), although in practice this principle is not always followed.

Clahsen et al. (2013) present a verbal description of both by-participants and by-items analyses:

> As regards the regular/irregular conditions, three-way ANOVAs for the factors Regularity (irregular/regular), Number (singular/plural) and Group (L2/L1) revealed significant main effects of Regularity ($F1(1,63) = 37.83$, $p < .001$; $F2(1,136) = 14.93$, $p < .001$) and Number ($F1(1,63) = 84.75$, $p < .001$; $F2(1,136) = 88.90$, $p < .001$) **in both the participant and item analyses**, and for Group ($F1(1,63) = 1.30$, $p = .259$; $F2(1,136) = 4.56$, $p < .05$) **in the item analysis only**, as well as an interaction of Regularity and Number ($F1(1,63) = 33.31$, $p < .001$; $F2(1,136) = 17.44$, $p < .001$).
>
> *(p. 18, emphasis added)*

Before running either *t*-tests or ANOVAs, it is important to check that the assumptions of these (parametric) tests are met. If assumptions regarding normality, skewness, homogeneity of variance, sphericity, or kurtosis are violated, the data can be transformed. See Vafaee et al. (2017) for a clear explanation of data transformation using several methods. Alternately, non-parametric tests may be used, most commonly the Mann-Whitney U-test (for independent measures) or the Wilcoxon test (for dependent measures) (e.g., Marsden, 2008).

6.5.3. Effect Sizes

When reporting the results of *t*-tests and ANOVAs, effect sizes should also be reported. Cohen's *d* is generally recommended and is most appropriate when comparing pairs of scores, whether within or between groups. However, classical and partial eta squared (η_p^2) are also frequently used, partially because they are automatically calculated by SPSS (see Norouzian & Plonsky, 2018, for discussion of partial and classical η^2). Effect sizes are useful because they indicate the size of the relationship between variables—and thus how important or meaningful the difference is—rather than simply whether there is likely to be a relationship or not (see, for example, Brysbaert & Stevens, 2018). Where there is a small number of participants, effect sizes may be useful for indicating whether an effect is present even if a difference is not statistically significant. They are also crucial for meta-analyses because they provide a standard metric, thus allowing results to be compared and combined across studies. The interpretation of effect sizes can involve the weighing of a variety of factors, but for second language studies, Plonsky and Oswald (2014) recommend the following general rules of thumb: small d = .40, medium d = .70, and large d = 1.00 for between-groups comparisons, and d = .60 small, d= 1.00 medium, and d = 1.40 large for pre-, post-, or within-group contrasts. For other considerations in interpreting effect sizes, see Plonsky and Oswald (2014). See Richardson (2011) for discussion on interpreting (partial) η^2, which expresses the amount (%) of variance in scores that can be accounted for by an independent variable such as target feature, (un)grammaticality, or group (e.g., NS vs. NNS). An example of a presentation of effect sizes (Table 6.6) comes from Tolentino and Tokowicz (2014, p. 298). Note that this study uses *d*-prime scores, which are discussed in Section 6.9.

6.5.4. Regressions

Judgment data are often subjected to various kinds of regression analyses in order to understand the relationship between the dependent variable and one or more

TABLE 6.6 Mean *d*-prime differences and effect sizes for the interaction between posttest, similarity, and instruction group (group comparison)

Posttest	*Contrast*	*Group*	*Mean Difference*	*Effect Size (Cohen's d)*
1	Unique vs. Dissimilar	R&S	1.03	.86
	Similar s. Dissimilar	Salience	.93	.64
2	Unique vs. Dissimilar	Salience	.78	.53
	Similar s. Dissimilar	Salience	.77	.54
3	Similar s. Dissimilar	Control	.99	.60

R&S= rule and salience

Source: From "Cross-language similarity modulates effectiveness of second language grammar instruction" by L. C. Tolentino & N. Tokowicz, 2014, *Language Learning*, *64*, p. 298. Published at the University of Michigan by Wiley. Reprinted by permission.

independent variables. Specifically, the goal is to determine the extent to which the variance in scores is accounted for by the independent variable. The most frequent use of this type of analysis has been with studies of critical period-type effects, where judgment data scores have been regressed to age of onset of acquisition (see Meulman, Wieling, Sprenger, Stowe, & Schmid, 2015, who used a mixed-effects logistic regression model). Yalçin and Spada (2016) collected aptitude data, oral production data, and judgment data on two grammatical structures (passive and past progressive). Their regression analysis is presented in Table 6.7 (p. 254).

To produce these results, the posttest scores were used as the criterion variable, and the aptitude test (here represented by LLAMA E [sound-symbol correspondence] a subcomponent of the LLAMA test developed by Meara, 2005) and pretest scores were predictor variables. The first step (indicated in the table) was to enter the pretest scores. The second step involved entering the aptitude scores. In Table 6.7, we see that the pretest scores were a significant predictor of posttest scores (β = 0.78). This predictor variable alone explained 61% of the variance on the posttest. The next part of the table shows that the aptitude subtest (LLAMA E) was not a significant predictor of the variance in the posttest scores, which is why the R^2 value of .61 remains unchanged even after adding the aptitude measure in step 2. For guidance on interpreting the R^2 values produced by regression models, see Plonsky and Ghanbar (2018).

6.5.5. Mixed-Effects Models

Schütze and Sprouse (2013) argue that best practice in dealing with judgment data is to use linear mixed-effects models when the data are numerical, as is the case with both magnitude estimation data or Likert-scale data, or to use logistic

TABLE 6.7 Summary of multiple regression analysis for aptitude components predicting passive GJT scores

	B	*SE B*	*β*
Step 1: Control Variable			
Constant	0.47	0.19	
Past Progressive GJT pretest	0.94	0.1	0.78**
Step 2: Aptitude Component			
Constant	.44	.2	
Past Progressive GJT pretest	.92	.1	0.77**
LLAMA E	0	0	.005

Source: From "Language aptitude and grammatical difficulty: An EFL classroom-based study" by S. Yalçin & N. Spada, 2016, *Studies in Second Language Acquisition*, 38, p. 254. Published by Cambridge University Press. Reprinted by permission.

** $p < 0.01$.

Note: R^2= .61 for Step 1, R^2 = .61 for Step 2 ($p < 0.01$).

mixed-effects models when data are non-numerical, as is the case with binary judgment tasks or preference tasks (where participants are asked to choose one sentence as better than another, e.g., *What do you think that John bought?* versus *What do you wonder whether John bought?*) (Schütze & Sprouse, 2013, p. 32). Nonetheless, even with binary choices, researchers often give an overall score that can then be treated as a continuous variable. Detailed discussions of statistical procedures go beyond the scope of this book; however, one should be aware of what is known as the "language-as-fixed-effect fallacy" (cf. Clark, 1973; Sprouse, 2013)—that is, the way data are understood in part depends on how one perceives those data. Are the sentences considered to be randomly selected from a larger set of sentences (random effects) or are they considered to represent the totality of the sentences tested (fixed effects)? Other effects of mixed-effects models are noted by Cunnings (2012, p. 372):

> Mixed-effects models are also robust against violations of sphericity and homoscedasticity (Quene & van den Bergh, 2004, 2008). Finally, SLA researchers are sometimes confronted with unbalanced datasets, as L2 learners can provide high numbers of missing responses in experimental studies. Mixed-effects models are robust against missing data, assuming that the data are missing at random, obviating the need to replace missing values using debatable imputation techniques (Quene & van den Bergh, 2004, 2008)

We raise these issues not to provide an answer but rather to make the reader aware of some of the issues involved in analyzing judgment data.

BOX 6.4 USING INFERENTIAL STATISTICS WITH JUDGMENT DATA

- For binary judgments, provide accuracy percentages and standard deviations for each category of sentences.
- For scalar judgments, provide mean ratings and standard deviations for each category of sentences.
- Check that assumptions are met before running statistical procedures. Report whether you have done so, and any transformations that you applied.
- Present descriptive data in a table along with text describing the statistical procedures and their results. Name any statistical procedures that are used.
- Consider running both a by-participants and by-items analysis of data; report both results.

- Report effect sizes for all statistical tests, whether or not their result is significant. Cohen's *d* is most appropriate for comparing pairs of group scores; (partial) eta squared (η_p^2) is used when comparing more than two sets of conditions or groups.
- Consider using a regression analysis to determine the relationship between dependent and one or more independent (predictor) variables.
- Consider a linear mixed-effect model so that both fixed and random effects can be specified.
- Whatever statistical analysis is used, familiarize yourself with standard statistical packages (e.g., *SPSS*, *R*) and the uses of such packages with linguistic data (e.g., Larson-Hall, 2016).

6.6. Reporting Individual Results

Averaging the performance of multiple participants can obscure patterns in the data. For example, imagine that there are 20 learners participating in a 20-item binary-choice judgment test. Half of the learners guess on every item, performing at chance level and getting half of them wrong (10/20, or 50%); the other half of the learners get every single item right (20/20, or 100%). The mean score of the group is 15/20 or 75%, which makes it appear that the learners have partial knowledge of the grammatical issue being examined. This conclusion would not, of course, truly reflect the nature of the individuals that make up this group of learners. While real results are rarely this clear, it is often advisable to examine the data to see whether individuals are patterning in distinct ways. One way to do this is to group participants into categories: those who accepted a majority of the items in a given category, those who rejected them, and those who had mixed results. Cuza (2013, p. 82) accomplished this through a table, reproduced as Table 6.8, in which judgment results are grouped by categories: accepted, unsure, and rejected. His 4-point scale consisted of the following: *odd*, *slightly odd*, *more or less fine*, *fine*. There were six matrix and six embedded sentences. To fall into the *accepted* category, a participant had to respond *fine* or *more or less fine* to three of the six sentences; to fall into the *rejected* category, a participant had to have two or less accepted responses. For the *unsure* category, they had to have three out of six accepted answers.

Ionin and Montrul (2010) present both group and individual results for a truth value judgment task (see Chapter 5) examining English plurals as generic or specific. Korean- and Spanish-speaking learners made binary judgments on sentences following a given context. There were 24 test items following eight stories (three per story), plus fillers. Eight sentences included bare plurals (e.g., *tigers*); eight included plurals with definite articles (e.g., *the tigers*), and eight included plurals with demonstratives (e.g., *these tigers*). When scoring the individual results,

TABLE 6.8 Acceptability judgment task: individual results within group per matrix and embedded ungrammatical questions

Group	*Accepted*	*Unsure*	*Rejected*
Heritage speakers			
Matrix	24% (4/17)	6% (1/17)	70% (12/17)
Embedded	76% (13/17)	12% (2/17)	12% (2/17)
Controls			
Matrix	0% (0/10)	10% (1/10)	90% (9/10)
Embedded	0% (0/10)	0% (0/10)	100% (10/10)

Source: From "Crosslinguistic influence at the syntax proper: Interrogative subject-verb inversion in heritage Spanish" by A. Cuza (2013), *International Journal of Bilingualism*, 17, p. 82. Published by Sage Journals. Reprinted by permission.

the authors divided participants into four different patterns, using six out of eight judgments per category as the criterion of target-like behavior. The first group, "target," included participants who were accurate in all three categories (bare plurals, definite plurals, and demonstrative plurals); that is, this group got at least six out of eight correct in each category. The second group, "definite generics," included participants who were accurate on six out of eight sentences with demonstrative plural and bare plurals, but had only five or fewer correct in the definite plural category. The third group, "bare specifics," were accurate on at least six out of eight sentences with demonstrative plurals and definite plural, but had five or fewer correct in the bare plural category. Finally, the authors included a group of "other" participants, who did not fit into the other patterns. They present the data regarding these patterns of behavior in figure form, as shown in Figure 6.1 (p. 899).

BOX 6.5 INDIVIDUAL RESULTS

- When working with groups, first inspect the results for potential patterns of individual behaviors. These patterns, if detected, should be reported separately from descriptive statistics for groups.
- Determine criteria for breaking participants into groups based on their performance and then report the numbers of participants in each group along with the criteria used to determine patterns.

6.7. Rasch Analysis

Although it is not commonly used, Tremblay (2005) makes a compelling argument for the use of a Rasch analysis using FACETS (Linacre, 1988) with judgment

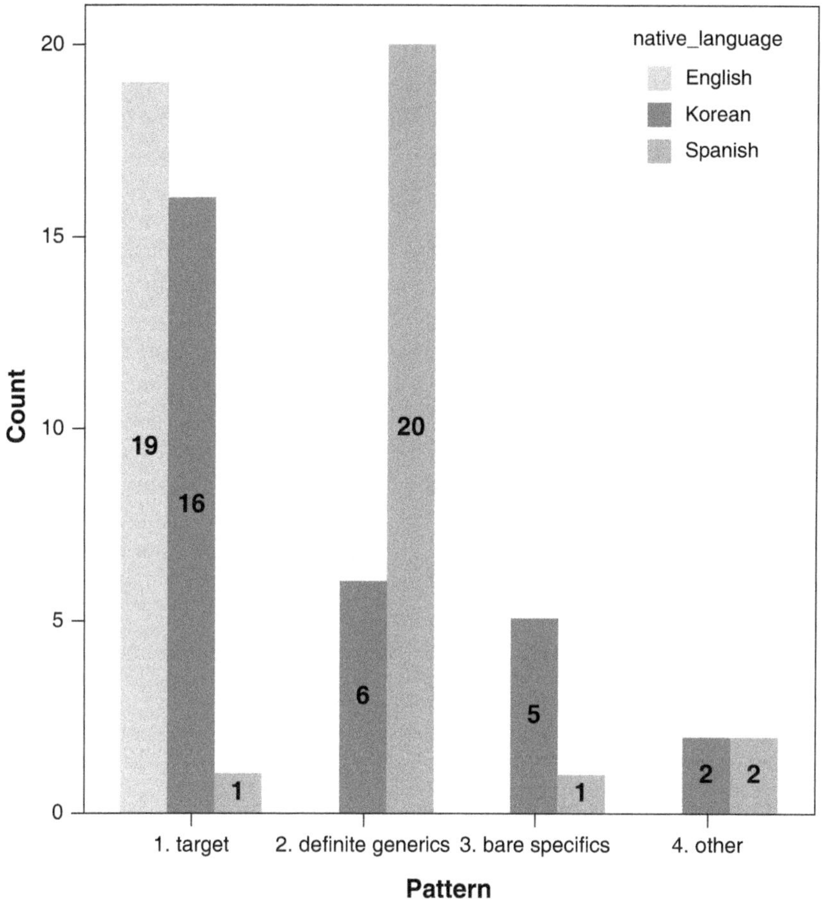

FIGURE 6.1 Individual participant patterns in the TVJT, by native language

Source: From "The role of L1 transfer in the interpretation of articles with definite plurals in L2 English" by T. Ionin & S. Montrul, *Language Learning, 60*, p. 899. Published at the University of Michigan by Wiley. Reprinted by permission.

data. FACETS is a Rasch measurement tool that is frequently used in language testing research to analyze rating data. In particular, the analysis can take into account internal consistency of ratings, for instance, whether participants may have a tendency to rate sentences as grammatical or ungrammatical, or whether certain items have a tendency to be rated high or low. This information can help pinpoint bad items in a judgment task or participants who should be removed from analysis. (Note, however, that a number of the goals of a Rasch analysis can be accomplished using *d*-prime scores, data transformations, or other methods outlined in this chapter.)

Tremblay's study involved 20 native speakers of English who took a computer-delivered timed judgment task. Sentences were judged on a 4-point scale ("perfect," "okay," "awkward," "horrible"); there was also a "no intuition" option. Figure 6.2 represents some of the results from her study. The leftmost column shows the logit scale, which represents the grammaticality of the sentences, while the rightmost column shows the actual rating scale used with the participants, with the two grammatical responses (*perfect* = *4*, *okay* = *3*) at the top and the two ungrammatical categories (*awkward* = *2*, *horrible* = *1*) at the bottom. It can be observed that the participants fall into a normal distribution, with a few participants (e.g., 118) judging sentences as more ungrammatical than the other participants, and a few participants (e.g., 103) judging sentences as more grammatical. Overall, though, the participants tended to judge sentences as more grammatical than ungrammatical, as can be observed from the fact that most participants' ratings are above the "0" mark, which is the division between the grammatical and ungrammatical items. The ratings of the types of sentences can be seen on this figure, as well. As expected, grammatical items are rated as grammatical, while ungrammatical items are rated as ungrammatical. However, two of the sentence types (factive and question) were rated more highly than expected, which can be observed in that they appear above 0 on the scale.

Figure 6.2 only reflects part of the analysis. For more detail, see Tremblay (2005).

BOX 6.6 RASCH ANALYSIS

- Determine if a Rasch analysis is a possible way to analyze and present your results.
- Some of the goals of a Rasch analysis can be accomplished using *d*-prime scores, data transformations, and the like.

6.8. Analyzing Likert Scale Data: *z*-Scores

Likert scale data are often analyzed very similarly to binary data, that is, by comparing mean scores. In this case, the scores do not reflect accuracy as they do with binary data, but rather a general idea of how acceptable participants find a group of sentences. However, it is not clear whether this is the most appropriate or complete analysis for these data, because points on the scale may have different meanings to the participants. For example, some participants may not consider any sentence "terrible" if they can get any meaning out of it at all, while others often consider a sentence terrible if it has even minor grammatical

```
--------------------------------------------------
|Measr|+Participants       |-Type|-Gramm|S.1   |
--------------------------------------------------
+   2 +                    +     +      +(4)   +
|     |                    |     |      |      |
|     |                    |     |      |      |
|     |                    |     |      |      |
|     | 103                |     |      |      |
|     |                    |     |      |      |
|     |                    |     | Grammatical |
|     | 120                |     |      |      |
|     | 102  114           |     |      | ---  |
|     | 116                |     |      |      |
+   1 +                    +     +      +      +
|     | 101  108  115      |     |      |      |
|     |                    |     |      |      |
|     | 105  110  111  117 |     |      |      |
|     | 119                | Factive    | 3    |
|     | 106  112  113      | Question   |      |
|     |                    |     |      |      |
|     | 104                |     |      |      |
|     | 107  109           |     |      |      |
|     |                    |     |      | ---  |
*   0 *                    *     *      *      *
|     | 118                |     |      |      |
|     |                    |     |      |      |
|     |                    |     |      |      |
|     |                    | Experimental 2    |
|     |                    |     |      |      |
|     |                    |     |      |      |
|     |                    | Control    |      |
|     |                    |     |      |      |
|     |                    |     |      |      |
+  -1 +                    +     +      +      +
|     |                    |     |      |      |
|     |                    |     |      | ---  |
|     |                    |     |      |      |
|     |                    |     | Ungrammatical
|     |                    |     |      |      |
|     |                    |     |      |      |
|     |                    |     |      |      |
|     |                    |     |      |      |
|     |                    |     |      |      |
+  -2 +                    +     +      +(1)   +
--------------------------------------------------
|Measr|+Participants       |-Type|-Gramm|S.1   |
--------------------------------------------------
```

FIGURE 6.2 Multi-faceted ruler along which the participants, sentence types, grammaticality, and ratings are represented

Source: From "Theoretical and methodological perspectives on the use of grammaticality judgment tasks in linguistic theory" by A. Tremblay, 2005, *Second Language Studies*, 24, p. 151. Reprinted by permission of A. Tremblay and J.D. Brown.

anomalies. Unfortunately, it is impossible to know how intervals are perceived by the respondent, even if clear instructions are provided (see discussion regarding clarity of instructions in Chapter 4.) In order to have a better picture of participants' responses to the scale while taking into account these individual differences, the data can be converted to *z*-scores. For an individual participant, a *z*-score with a positive value is higher than his or her mean rating, while a negative value is lower. Any values that are one standard deviation higher or lower than the mean represent more extreme responses, assuming that the results are normally distributed.

Though not common in published second language studies utilizing judgment data, the use of *z*-scores is recommended in general linguistics (Schütze & Sprouse, 2013), with example studies including Casasanto, Hofmeister, and Sag (2010), Hofmeister et al. (2015), and Perek and Goldberg (2017). Cowart (1997) refers to the use of *z*-scores as a "way to minimize difference in the way informants use a scale" (p. 114). Over 25 years later, we find the same point made by Schütze and Sprouse (2013), who are more forceful in their proclamation, stating that "many researchers, including us, believe that the *z*-score transformation should be used routinely" when Likert scales have been used (p. 43). They are careful to point out that not everyone agrees, in particular because Likert-scale data are not continuous, whereas *z*-scores do represent continuous data. *z*-scores can be used with parametric analyses that assume continuous data, and it is reasonable to treat Likert-scale data as continuous for the purposes of analysis.

In a study of language impairment, Miller, Leonard, and Finneran (2008) display results in terms of *z*-scores in tabular form. There are three groups in their study: normal language development (NLD), specific language impairment (SLI), and nonspecific language impairment (NLI). Their data, which include *z*-score results, are shown in Table 6.9.

TABLE 6.9 Mean (SD) participant data by group

Group	*Age in Years*[a]	*Mother's Education in Years*[b]	*Performance IQ*	*Language Composite z-Score*[c]
NLD	15.8 (0.3)	13.7 (2.2)	102 (10)	-.18 (0.76)
SLI	15.9 (0.4)	12.9 (1.5)	98 (9)	-1.54 (0.35)
NLI	15.9 (0.4)	12.6 (1.5)	76 (6)	-1.76 (0.61)

Source: From "Grammaticality judgments in adolescents with and without language impairment" by K. Miller, L. Leonard & D. Finneran, 2008, *International Journal of Language Communication*, 43, p. 352. Published by Wiley. Reprinted by permission.

a Age data missing for one participant in NLD group;
b Mother's education data missing for two participants in NLD group, one participant in NLI group;
c *z*-scores based on standardization of entire longitudinal sample of 527 participants.

Another way of displaying *z*-score results is through bar graphs. Casasanto et al. (2010), in a study that *inter alia* investigates processing difficulties in relation to acceptability judgments describe their use of *z*-scores as follows:

> we computed z-scores for each subject on the basis of all data in the experimental data set (except practice items), including fillers. This reduces the impact of varying uses of the interval scale by subjects. Finally, we excluded data points with z-scores more than 2.5 standard deviations from the mean for each participant. For Experiment I, this outlier removal process affected 2.0% of the data. The resulting z-scores constitute the data on which we conducted statistical analyses.
>
> *(p. 226)*

In their study, they were concerned with the hierarchical distance between subject and object and the subcategorizing verb. The manipulation involved insertion of a relative clause between subject and verb and placing the object after the verb or before the verb by relativizing that noun. This resulted in four conditions: 1) *The nurse from the clinic supervised the administrator who scolded the medic while a patient was brought into the emergency room* [short-short], 2) *The nurse who was from the clinic supervised the administrator who scolded the medic while a patient was brought into the emergency room* [long-short], 3) *The administrator who the nurse from the clinic supervised scolded the medic while a patient was brought into the emergency room,* [short-long], and 4) *The administrator who the nurse who was from the clinic supervised scolded the medic while a patient was brought into the emergency room* [long-long]. Participants rated the magnitude of acceptability. Their *z*-score results are displayed in Figure 6.3.

With binary responses, *d*-prime analysis, which uses *z*-scores, is more commonly used than *z*-scores alone (see Section 6.9).

Another potential issue with analyzing scalar data is that the intervals between points may vary. For instance, a participant may consider there to be only a slight difference between a "terrible" rating and a "quite bad" rating, but a big difference between "quite bad" and "okay." In other words, the scale is an ordinal scale. However, parametric statistics such as ANOVA require an interval scale, that is, one in which the difference between scores is meaningful and standardized (similar to points on a thermometer). One way that some researchers get around this issue is to collapse responses on the "accept" versus "reject" side of the scale (e.g., "terrible" and "quite bad" are considered rejections; "pretty good" and "perfect" are acceptances) and then treat the data as binary responses. However, the downside to this practice is that it eliminates the fine-grained information regarding gradience of grammaticality (see Tremblay, 2005, p. 147). A better solution is to transform the data by converting them into natural logarithmic values, placing them on a linear interval scale rather than an ordinal scale and thus allowing the

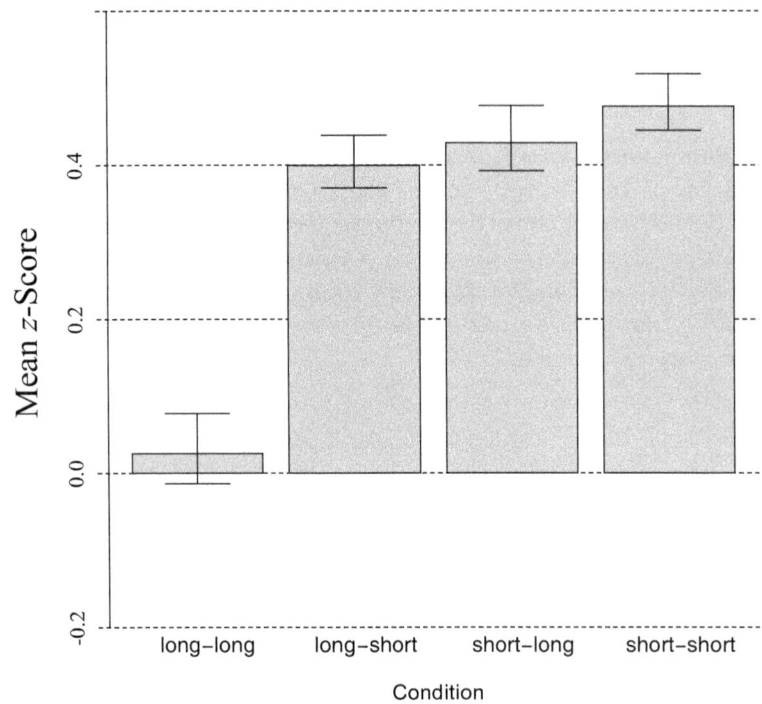

FIGURE 6.3 Acceptability z-scores for experiment I. Error bars show (+/−) one standard error

Source: "Understanding acceptability judgments: Additivity and working memory effects" by L. Casasanto, P. Hofmeister & I. Sag. *Cognitive Science Society*. p. 26.

use of t-tests or ANOVAs. This can be done with most statistical packages. Pae, Schanding, Kwon, and Lee (2014) provide the following justification for using a natural logarithmic scale:

> An initial normality check showed that the data were positively skewed. In order to normalize the data to satisfy the normality assumption, a data transformation was performed. Furthermore, since raw scores and percentages were sample dependent (i.e., ordinal level measures) and could be distorted on both ends of the scoring continuum, the data were placed on a linear interval scale by converting the data into natural logarithmic values. The logarithmic scale was used in the process of maximum likelihood estimation. This was done because a difference of ten score points at different locations on the scoring continuum had different meanings.
>
> *(p. 196)*

> **BOX 6.7 USING STANDARDIZED SCORES**
>
> - Best practice is to transform Likert-scale data to *z*-scores to better take into account individual differences in using the Likert scale.
> - Consider converting Likert data to natural logarithmic values to compensate for the fact the intervals between original data points may vary.
> - Use parametric tests with *z*-scores, although recognize that Likert-scale data may not represent continuous data.

6.9. Binary Judgments: *d*-Prime Scores

For binary judgments, some recent research has employed *d'* (*d*-prime) analyses, originally used in signal detection research (see Macmillan & Creelman, 2004). Analysis with *d*-prime takes into account response bias, that is, the tendency of some individuals to provide a disproportionately large number of positive or negative responses on a judgment task. The *d*-prime score provides a better measure of the ability of participants to discriminate between grammatical and ungrammatical stimuli by compensating for response patterns. The *d*-prime is calculated using *z*-scores. Generally, high *d*-prime values indicate good discrimination; values of 0 or below indicate poor discrimination. In reporting results, accuracy scores and standard deviations are typically presented along with the *d*-prime scores and standard deviations. Additionally, *d*-prime scores can be used with *t*-tests and ANOVAs. For examples of *d*-prime scores used in L2 judgment task research, see Morgan-Short, Sanz, Steinhauer, and Ullman (2010), Rebuschat and Williams (2012), Tagarelli, Ruiz, Vega, and Rebuschat (2016) and Tolentino and Tokowicz (2014). For example, Tagarelli et al. focused on the interaction of three variables: exposure conditions, syntactic complexity, and individual differences. Table 6.10, taken from their study, shows how *d'* scores are displayed. Figure 6.4, also from Tagarelli et al., shows a boxplot display of *d'* performance (see Larson-Hall & Herrington, 2009 for arguments regarding visual presentation of data).

It is to be noted that *d*-prime scores can also be calculated for confidence ratings and source ratings.

> **BOX 6.8 *D*-PRIME**
>
> - Analysis with *d*-prime is a good choice for judgment tasks because it takes into account response bias.
> - *t*-tests and ANOVAs can be used with *d*-prime scores.

TABLE 6.10 Accuracy (%) and *d'* scores on the GJT for each group overall and according to complexity

	Incidental				*Instructed*			
	Accuracy		*d'*		*Accuracy*		*d'*	
	M	*SD*	*M*	*SD*	*M*	*SD*	*M*	*SD*
All	55.53	9.69	0.19**	0.32	65.33	15.65	0.63****	0.64
Simple	60.60	13.49	0.42***	0.64	75.69	17.70	1.00****	0.81
Complex 1	60.00	11.82	0.04	0.49	63.12	18.77	0.46*	0.85
Complex 2	56.00	19.20	0.28	0.74	63.53	25.00	0.64***	0.92

Source: From "Variability in second language learning: The roles of individual differences, learning conditions, and linguistic complexity" by K. Tagarelli, S. Ruiz, J. Vega & P. Rebuschat, 2016, *Studies in Second Language Acquisition, 38*, p. 304. Published by Cambridge University Press. Reprinted by permission.

Significance from chance: *p = .07, * $p < .05$, **$p < .01$, *** $p < .005$, and **** $p < .001$

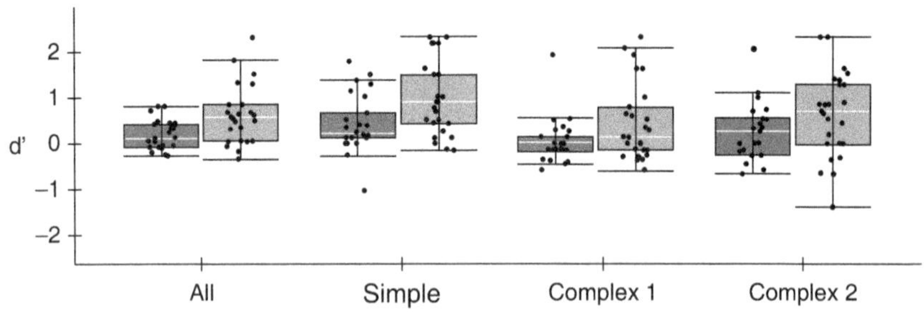

FIGURE 6.4 Boxplots of *d*-prime performance for all sentences, and for each sentence group. Error bars represent standard deviation. Dark gray boxes = incidental condition; light gray boxes = instructed condition

Source: From "Variability in second language learning: The roles of individual differences, learning conditions, and linguistic complexity" by K. Tagarelli, S. Ruiz, J. Vega & P. Rebuschat, 2016, *Studies in Second Language Acquisition, 38*, p. 305. Published by Cambridge University Press. Reprinted by permission.

6.10. Analyzing Magnitude Estimation Scores

Magnitude estimation allows an open-ended rating system in which participants can assign their own values to sentences of varying acceptability. Participants begin by assigning a score (*modulus*) to a reference or baseline sentence (*standard*), and then are asked to rate all target sentences as a proportion of the value they assigned to the standard (Schütze & Sprouse, 2013). The scales that participants use may vary widely; thus, in order to perform analysis on the results, a common scale needs to be used for all participants. To accomplish this, each participant's responses are rescaled, typically to a 0-to-100 scale (although any scale could be used as long as it is uniform among participants). For example, to convert her participants' scores to a 10-point scale, Yuan (1995) used the following formula:

Converted score = 10 x (Individual Raw number – minimum score / maximum score – minimum score).

Each rating is then divided by the value that participants assign to the modulus (benchmark) sentence. Another option is to first divide each rating by the value applied to the modulus sentence and then apply a logarithmic transformation to the data, which normalizes it and brings it to a common scale (see Kraš, 2011). Means for groups and conditions are calculated, generally using geometric means instead of mathematical means (see Bard et al., 1996; Hopp, 2010). Standard procedures for *t*-tests or ANOVAs are then usually carried out.

BOX 6.9 MAGNITUDE ESTIMATION

- Magnitude estimation is useful to elicit scalar, fine-grained judgments.
- Rescale participants' responses to a common scale, the most common being either a *z*-transformation or a logarithmic transformation.

6.11. Using Response Time Data

In some experimental designs, the amount of time participants take to make a decision on each item is measured. These time measurements provide information about the amount of cognitive resources it took to make a decision. Generally, it is assumed that when the response times are higher, more cognitive resources were necessary to make the decision. Usually the amount of time is not open-ended; that is, there is typically a cutoff point for making a decision, for instance four seconds after presentation of the stimuli. If a participant fails to respond during this time, the trial is aborted and the next sentence appears. These cases are often considered inaccurate responses and included with them, but they may also be removed from analysis. The percentage of aborted trials should be reported. When writing up a study, information regarding response times is presented along with accuracy scores or mean rating scores, as was the case in a study by Knightley, Jun, Oh, and Au (2003), partially reproduced in Table 6.11, which shows only the judgment task results.

While the Knightley et al. (2003) study combined responses to grammatical and ungrammatical items, Della Putta (2016) analyzes grammatical and ungrammatical sentences separately and presents the data in separate tables, as can be seen in Tables 6.12 and 6.13, where descriptive statistics are presented for reaction times to make judgments on sentences by Spanish-speaking learners of Italian. These tables display responses to sentences with the prepositional accusative (PA). −PA sentences are grammatical in Italian; +PA sentences are ungrammatical in Italian.

TABLE 6.11 Participants' performance on Spanish morphosyntax assessment tasks (only judgment data are presented here)

Measure	*Native Speakers*	*Childhood Overhearers*	*Typical Late L2 Learners*
Grammaticality judgment percentage correct	91.8[a] (0.97)	63.6[b] (1.6)	62.5[b] (2.6)
Reaction time (ms)	1201 [a] (124)	2661[b] (283)	1936 [a] (307)

Source: From "Production benefits of childhood overhearing" by L. Knightley, S.-A. Jun, J. Oh & T. Au, 2013, *Journal of the Acoustical Society of America, 114*, p. 471. Reprinted by permission.

The table indicates the mean percentage correct unless otherwise specified. Standard errors are given in parentheses. Within a row, means with different superscripts were reliably different from each other according to Tukey's HSD test, p < 0.01. Numbers with the same superscript were not reliably different from each other.

TABLE 6.12 Descriptive statistics of −PA RTs

	Group A (n = 35)		*Group B (n = 33)*	
	m	*SD*	*m*	*SD*
Pretest	3,561.93	568.09	3689.21	504.17
Posttest	4,277.8	720.02	3,486.37	842.64
Delayed posttest	3,952.67	646.61	3,555.42	457.27

Source: From "The effects of textual enhancement on the acquisition of two nonparallel grammatical features by Spanish-speaking learners of Italian" by P. Della Putta, 2016, *Studies in Second Language Acquisition, 38*, p. 231. Published by Cambridge University Press. Reprinted by permission.

Note: RT values range from 0 to 6,000 m. m = mean

TABLE 6.13 Descriptive statistics of +PA RTs

	Group A (n = 35)		*Group B (n = 33)*	
	m	*SD*	*m*	*SD*
Pretest	3,310.81	500.83	3,249.78	521
Posttest	3,453.11	509.43	3,247.72	377.26
Delayed posttest	3296.45	451.09	3,471.67	461.75

Source: From "The effects of textual enhancement on the acquisition of two nonparallel grammatical features by Spanish-speaking learners of Italian" by P. Della Putta, 2016, *Studies in Second Language Acquisition, 38*, p. 232. Published by Cambridge University Press. Reprinted by permission.

Note: RT values range from 0 to 6,000 m. m = mean

In some cases, it may be desirable to only include response times on correctly answered items in response time analyses. The reasoning is that the response time can tell you about the resources it took to make a decision when the answer was accurate. When the answer is inaccurate, it is not clear what the participants were doing or how they parsed the sentence, which makes it harder to interpret the response time.

An initial step in preparing response time data for analysis is removing outliers: any response times that are 2–3 standard deviations from the participant's mean (higher and lower) are typically eliminated, although there are differing views on when this should be done (cf. Bakker & Wicherts, 2014 for a useful paper on handling outliers in psychological research). There are two important reasons for the elimination of outliers. First, it is possible that something unusual happened during those responses (e.g., a finger slipping, a sneeze). Second, eliminating outliers helps to ensure statistical robustness. Another way to eliminate responses that are too fast (i.e., a very low response time) is to use a fixed minimum amount, such as 750 ms, for a sentence (see Jiang, 2012). The reasoning here is that the participant would not have had time to fully process the material and therefore must have responded too quickly for some reason. The percentage of data that is trimmed during these processes should be reported.

Once response time data are cleaned, they will often be reported along with accuracy rates. There is no one way to interpret differences in response times on items. Increased response times may be taken as a sign of difficulty and confusion or, somewhat paradoxically, as an increased sensitivity to grammatical structures or grammatical violations.

BOX 6.10 RESPONSE TIME DATA WITH JUDGMENTS

- It is common to trim the data by eliminating outliers 2–3 standard deviations from the mean. A lower threshold for reaction time data may also be set to ensure that participants have had time to process the material before giving a response.
- Report the percentage of data that is trimmed during the process of cleaning the data.
- Consider whether you want to report response times only for sentences that are correctly judged. This will depend on your research question and your interpretation of incorrectly judged sentences.

6.12. Using Judgment Data Results in Conjunction With Other Measures

Earlier in the history of the field, judgment tasks were frequently used as the central or only measure in a study. In recent years, it has been more widely recognized that different tasks tap into different aspects of participants' knowledge and ability, and judgment tasks tend to be used in combination with other measures. As Table 6.14 shows, beginning with the 1970s until the current decade, the

TABLE 6.14 Percentage of studies using judgment data in conjunction with other measures

Decade	*Percentage Using Measures in Addition to Judgment Data*
1970s (n=3)	33%
1980s (n=10)	40%
1990s (n=53)	43%
2000s (n=90)	61%
2010s (n=142)	68%

percentage of studies that use additional measures in conjunction with a standard judgment task has more than doubled (based on data analyzed in Plonsky et al., in press).

This trend suggests that it is generally seen as valuable to use tasks that tap into knowledge and processes that judgment tasks may miss. For example, because judgment tasks are a measure of receptive knowledge, they are often combined with productive tasks such as picture description, interviews, narration tasks, etc. Additionally, because judgment tasks are generally offline (in the sense that we cannot see the decision-making process in action, but rather only see the result of a decision), they are often combined with online measures such as eye-tracking or self-paced reading (see Godfroid et al., 2015). The results from the various measures may converge to convey a consistent estimation of participants' knowledge and abilities with a certain structure, or they may diverge, in which case it may be that learners have incomplete or partial knowledge or ability with a particular structure.

With some studies there is a desire to determine whether there are relationships between performance on different tasks. This approach is best exemplified in a study by Ellis (2005) that investigated which task types tapped into L2 learners' implicit vs. explicit knowledge. In this study, participants completed five tasks, including both a timed and untimed judgment task, an oral imitation test, an oral narration test, and a metalinguistic knowledge test. Through a principal component analysis, Ellis found that participant performance on the timed judgment task (along with oral imitation and narration) was associated with implicit L2 knowledge, while performance on the untimed judgment task (and metalinguistic knowledge test) was associated with explicit L2 knowledge. Ellis' approach has been replicated by several studies since, using both exploratory (e.g., Erçetin & Alptekin, 2013) and confirmatory (e.g., Bowles, 2011; Zhang, 2015) factor analyses.

BOX 6.11 JUDGMENT DATA WITH OTHER MEASURES

- Judgment tasks are limited in the type of information that they reveal about learners' knowledge about their L2. Additional complementary tasks are often useful.
- Consider including other tasks, including production tasks, online tasks, or tasks that encourage the use of implicit knowledge, in your study along with judgment tasks. Make sure you carefully consider the purpose of each task and what you are hoping each task will reveal about L2 knowledge.

6.13. Conclusion

In this chapter, we have presented some basic information about ways to analyze judgment data. It was our intent to cover only the most commonly used analyses of judgment data and not to present an exhaustive list of the various approaches and statistical procedures that have been used. As with any research, the specific analysis will depend on the design of the task and the research questions being addressed. There are numerous books in the field of second language acquisition that address research methodology and design (e.g., Mackey & Gass, 2016; Phakiti, 2014; Dörnyei, 2007) as well as books that provide in-depth information about tools of analysis and computer programs that help with that analysis (e.g., Larson-Hall, 2016). We urge readers to avail themselves of these resources as they make important decisions regarding data analysis.

Note

1. It is generally no longer considered best practice to replace scores with the mean in this way (Plonsky, personal communication, July 18, 2018) because it may artificially reduce variance in scores. Rather, it is better for problematic items to be removed from analysis.

REFERENCES

Abrahamsson, N. (2012). Age of onset and nativelike L2 ultimate attainment of morpho-syntactic and phonetic intuition. *Studies in Second Language Acquisition, 34*, 187–214. https://doi.org/10.1017/S0272263112000022

Akakura, M. (2012). Evaluating the effectiveness of explicit instruction on implicit and explicit L2 knowledge. *Language Teaching Research, 16*, 9–37. https://doi.org/10.1177/1362168811423339

Akmajian, A., & Heny, F. (1975). *An introduction to the principles of transformational syntax*. Cambridge, MA: MIT Press.

Alexiadou, A., & Stavrakaki, S. (2006). Clause structure and verb movement in a Greek—English speaking bilingual patient with Broca's aphasia: Evidence from adverb placement. *Brain and Language, 96*, 207–220. https://doi.org/10.1016/j.bandl.2005.04.006

Alexopoulou, T., & Keller, F. (2007). Locality, cyclicity and resumption: At the interface between the grammar and the human sentence processor. *Language, 83*, 110–160. https://doi.org/10.1353/lan.2007.0001

Alptekin, C., Erçetin, G., & Özemir, O. (2014). Effects of variations in reading span task design on the relationship between working memory capacity and second language reading. *The Modern Language Journal, 98*, 536–552. https://doi.org/10.1111/modl.12089

Andringa, S., & Curcic, M. (2015). How explicit knowledge affects online L2 processing. *Studies in Second Language Acquisition, 37*, 237–268. https://doi.org/10.1017/S0272263115000017

Ard, J., & Gass, S. (1987). Lexical constraints on syntactic acquisition. *Studies in Second Language Acquisition, 9*, 233–252. https://doi.org/10.1017/S0272263100000498

Athanasopoulos, P. (2006). Effects of the grammatical representation of number on cognition in bilinguals. *Bilingualism: Language and Cognition, 9*, 89–96. https://doi.org/10.1017/S1366728905002397

Ayoun, D. (2014). The acquisition of future temporality by L2 French learners. *Journal of French Language Studies, 24*, 181–202. https://doi.org/10.1017/S0959269513000185

Baayen, R. H. (2008). *Analyzing linguistic data: A practical introduction to statistics using R*. Cambridge: Cambridge University Press.

Baddeley, A. (2003). Working memory: Looking back and looking forward. *Nature Reviews Neuroscience, 4*, 829–839. https://doi.org/10.1038/nrn1201

Bakker, M., & Wickerts, J. (2014). Outlier removal and the relation with reporting errors and quality of psychological research. *PLOS One, 7*. https://doi.org/10.1371/journal.pone.0103360

Bard, E. G., Robertson, D., & Sorace, A. (1996). Magnitude estimation of linguistic acceptability. *Language, 72*, 32–68. https://doi.org/10.2307/416793

Bardovi-Harlig, K., & Dörnyei, Z. (1998). Do language learners recognize pragmatic violations? Pragmatic versus grammatical awareness in instructed L2 learning. *TESOL Quarterly, 32*, 233–259. https://doi.org/10.2307/3587583

Barrios, A., & Bernardo, A. (2012). The acquisition of case marking by L1 Chabacano and L1 Cebuano learners of L2 Filipino: Influence of actancy structure on transfer. *Language and Linguistics, 13*, 499–521. Retrieved from www.ling.sinica.edu.tw/Files/LL/Docments/Journals/13.3/j2012_3_05_0001.pdf

Batterink, L., & Neville, H. (2013). Implicit and explicit second language training recruit common neural mechanisms for syntactic processing. *Journal of Cognitive Neuroscience, 25*, 936–951. https://doi.org/10.1162/jocn_a_00354

Bauer, H. (1991). Sore finger items in multiple-choice tests. *System, 19*, 453–458. https://doi.org/10.1016/0346-251X(91)90025-K

Bautista, M. L. S. (2004). The verb in Philippine English: A preliminary analysis of modal *would*. *World Englishes, 23*, 113–128. https://doi.org/10.1111/j.1467-971X.2004.00338.x

Bever, T., & Carroll, J. (1981). On some continuous properties in language. In T. Myers, J. Laver, & J. Anderson (Eds.), *The cognitive representation of speech* (pp. 225–233). Amsterdam, The Netherlands: North-Holland.

Bialystok, E. (1978). A theoretical model of second language learning. *Language Learning, 28*, 69–83. https://doi.org/10.1111/j.1467 1770.1978.tb00305.x

Bialystok, E. (1979). Explicit and implicit judgements of L2 grammaticality. *Language Learning, 29*, 81–103. https://doi.org/10.1111/j.1467-1770.1979.tb01053.x

Bialystok, E. (1997). The structure of age: In search of barriers to second language acquisition. *Second Language Research, 13*, 116–137. https://doi.org/10.1191/026765897677670241

Bianchi, G. (2013). Gender in Italian—German bilinguals: A comparison with German L2 learners of Italian. *Bilingualism: Language and Cognition, 16*, 538–557. doi:10.1017/S1366728911000745

Birdsong, D. (1992). Ultimate attainment in second language acquisition. *Language, 68*, 706–755. https://doi.org/10.2307/416851

Birdsong, D., & Flege, J. (2001). *Regular-irregular dissociations in L2 acquisition of English morphology*. BUCLD 25: Proceedings of the 25th Annual Boston University Conference on Language Development (pp. 123–132). Boston, MA: Cascadilla Press.

Bley-Vroman, R. (1983). The comparative fallacy in interlanguage studies: The case of systematicity. *Language Learning, 33*, 1–17. https://doi.org/10.1111/j.1467-1770.1983.tb00983.x

Bley-Vroman, R. (1990). The logical problem of foreign language learning. *Linguistic Analysis, 20*, 3–49. https://doi.org/10.1017/CBO9781139524544.005

Bley-Vroman, R., & Chaudron, C. (1990). Second language processing of subordinate clauses and anaphora: First language and universal influences: A review of Flynn's research. *Language Learning, 40*, 245–285. https://doi.org/10.1111/j.1467-1770.1990.tb01335.x

Bley-Vroman, R., Felix, S. W., & Ioup, G. L. (1988). The accessibility of Universal Grammar in adult language learning. *Second Language Research, 4*, 1–32. https://doi.org/10.1177/026765838800400101

Bley-Vroman, R., & Yoshinaga, N. (2000). The acquisition of multiple wh-questions by high-proficiency non-native speakers of English. *Second Language Research*, *16*, 3–26. https://doi.org/10.1191/026765800676857467

Bloomfield, L. (1935). Linguistic aspects of science. *Philosophy of Science*, *2*, 499–517. https://doi.org/10.1086/286392

Bordag, D., & Pechmann, T. (2007). Factors influencing L2 gender processing. *Bilingualism: Language and Cognition*, *10*, 299–314. https://doi.org/10.1017/S1366728907003082

Borgonovo, C., de Garavito, J. B., & Prévost, P. (2015). Mood selection in relative clauses: Interfaces and variability. *Studies in Second Language Acquisition*, *37*, 33–69. https://doi.org/10.1017/S0272263114000321

Bowles, M. (2011). Measuring implicit and explicit linguistic knowledge: What can heritage language learners contribute? *Studies in Second Language Acquisition*, *33*, 247–271. https://doi.org/10.1017/S0272263110000756

Branigan, H., & Pickering, M. (2017). An experimental approach to linguistic representation. *Behavioral and Brain Sciences*, *40*. https://doi.org/10.1017/S0140525X16002028

Bresnan, J. (1977). Variables in the theory of transformations. In P. Culicover, T. Wasow, & A. Akmajian (Eds.), *Formal syntax* (pp. 157–196). New York, NY: Academic Press.

Bresnan, J. (2007). Is syntactic knowledge probabilistic? Experiments with the English dative alternation. In S. Featherston & W. Sternefeld (Eds.), *Roots: Linguistics in search of its evidential base* (pp. 75–96). Berlin: Mouton de Gruyter.

Bresnan, J., & Ford, M. (2010). Predicting syntax: Processing dative constructions in American and Australian varieties of English. *Language*, *86*, 168–213. https://doi.org/10.1353/lan.0.0189

Bruhn de Garavito, J. B. (2011). Subject/object asymmetries in the grammar of bilingual and monolingual Spanish speakers: Evidence against connectionism. *Linguistic Approaches to Bilingualism*, *1*, 111–148. https://doi.org/10.1075/lab.1.2.01bru

Bruhn de Garavito, J. B., & Valenzuela, E. (2008). Eventive and stative passives in Spanish L2 acquisition: A matter of aspect. *Bilingualism: Language and Cognition*, *11*, 323–336. https://doi.org/10.1017/S1366728908003556

Brysbaert, M., & Stevens, M. (2018). Power analysis and effect size in mixed effects models: A tutorial. *Journal of Cognition*, *1*. https://doi.org/10.5334/joc.10

Carroll, J., Bever, T., & Pollack, C. (1981). The non-uniqueness of linguistic intuitions. *Language*, *57*, 368–383. https://doi.org/10.2307/413695

Casasanto, L., Hofmeister, P., & Sag, I. (2010). Understanding acceptability judgments: Additivity and working memory effects. *Cognitive Science Society*, 224–229. Retrieved from http://repository.essex.ac.uk/4244/

Chaudron, C. (1983). Research on metalinguistic judgments: A review of theory, methods, and results. *Language Learning*, *33*, 343–377. https://doi.org/10.1111/j.1467-1770.1983.tb00546.x

Cho, J. (2017). The acquisition of different types of definite noun phrases in L2 English. *International Journal of Bilingualism*, *21*, 367–382. https://doi.org/10.1177/1367006916629577

Cho, J., & Slabakova, R. (2017). A feature-based contrastive approach to the L2 Acquisition of Specificity. *Applied Linguistics*, *38*, 318–339. https://doi.org/10.1093/applin/amv029

Chomsky, N. (1957). *Syntactic structures*. The Hague: Mouton.

Chomsky, N. (1961). Some methodological remarks on generative grammar. *Word*, *17*, 219–239.

Chomsky, N. (1965). *Aspects of the theory of syntax*. Cambridge, MA: MIT Press.

Chomsky, N., & Lasnik, H. (1977). Filters and control. *Linguistic Inquiry*, *8*, 425–508.

Chomsky, N., & Miller, G. A. (1963). Introduction to the formal analysis of natural languages. In R. D. Lace, R. R. Bush, & E. Galanter (Eds.), *Handbook of mathematical psychology Volume II* (pp. 269–321). New York, NY: Wiley-Blackwell.

Clahsen, H., Balkhair, L., Schutter, J. S., & Cunnings, I. (2013). The time course of morphological processing in a second language. *Second Language Research, 29*, 7–31. https://doi.org/10.1177/0267658312464970

Clark, H. (1973). The language-as-fixed-effect fallacy: A critique of language statistics in psychology research. *Journal of Verbal Learning and Verbal Behavior, 12*, 335–359.

Conroy, M., & Cupples, L. (2010). We could have loved and lost, or we never could have love at all: Syntactic misanalysis in L2 sentence processing. *Studies in Second Language Acquisition, 32*, 523–552. https://doi.org/10.1017/S0272263110000252

Conway, A. R., Kane, M. J., Bunting, M. F., Hambrick, D. Z., Wilhelm, O., & Engle, R. W. (2005). Working memory span tasks: A methodological review and user's guide. *Psychonomic Bulletin & Review, 12*, 769–786. https://doi.org/10.3758/BF03196772

Cook, V. (2003). The poverty-of-the-stimulus argument and structure-dependency in L2 users of English. *International Review of Applied Linguistics in Language Teaching, 41*, 201–221. https://doi.org/10.1515/iral.2003.009

Corder, S. P. (1973). The elicitation of interlanguage. *Errata: Papers in Error Analysis*, 36–48.

Cormier, K., Schembri, A., Vinson, D., & Orfanidou, E. (2012). First language acquisition differs from second language acquisition in prelingually deaf signers: Evidence from sensitivity to grammaticality judgement in British Sign Language. *Cognition, 124*, 50–65. https://doi.org/10.1016/j.cognition.2012.04.003

Coughlin, C. E., & Tremblay, A. (2013). Proficiency and working memory based explanations for nonnative speakers' sensitivity to agreement in sentence processing. *Applied Psycholinguistics, 34*, 615–646. https://doi.org/10.1017/S0142716412000616

Cowan, R., & Hatasa, Y. A. (1994). Investigating the validity and reliability of native speaker and second-language learner judgments about sentences. In E. Tarone, S. M. Gass, & A. Cohen (Eds.), *Research methodology in second language acquisition* (pp. 287–302). Hillsdale, NJ: Lawrence Erlbaum Associates.

Cowart, W. (1997). *Experimental syntax: Applying objective methods to sentence judgments.* Thousand Oaks, CA: Sage.

Cox, J. G., & Sanz, C. (2015). Deconstructing PI for the ages: Explicit instruction vs. practice in young and older adult bilinguals. *International Review of Applied Linguistics in Language Teaching, 53*, 225–248. https://doi.org/10.1515/iral-2015-0011

Culbertson, J., & Gross, S. (2009). Are linguists better subjects? *The British Journal of the Philosophy of Science, 60*, 721–736. https://doi.org/10.1093/bjps/axp032

Culicover, P. (2013). *Grammar and complexity: Language at the interface of competence and performance.* Oxford: Oxford University Press.

Cunnings, I. (2012). An overview of mixed-effects statistical models for second language researchers. *Second Language Research, 28*, 369–382. https://doi.org/10.1177/0267658312443651

Cuza, A. (2013). Crosslinguistic influence at the syntax proper: Interrogative subject-verb inversion in heritage Spanish. *International Journal of Bilingualism, 17*, 71–96. https://doi.org/10.1177/1367006911432619

Cuza, A., & Frank, J. (2015). On the role of experience and age-related effects: Evidence from the Spanish CP. *Second Language Research, 31*, 3–28. https://doi.org/10.1177/0267658314532939

D'Arcy, A. (2017). *Discourse-pragmatic variation in context: Eight-hundred years of LIKE*. Amsterdam, The Netherlands: John Benjamins.

Dabrowska, E. (2010). Naive v. expert intuitions: An empirical study of acceptability judgments. *The Linguistic Review*, *27*, 1–23. https://doi.org/10.1515/tlir.2010.001

de Graaff, R. (1997). The "Experanto" experiment: Effects of explicit instruction on second language acquisition. *Studies in Second Language Acquisition*, *19*, 249–276.

DeKeyser, R. (2000). The robustness of critical period effects in second language acquisition. *Studies in Second Language Acquisition*, *22*, 499–533. https://doi.org/10.2307/44486933

DeKeyser, R. (2007). *Practice in a second language: Perspectives from applied linguistics and cognitive psychology*. Cambridge: Cambridge University Press.

DeKeyser, R., Alfi-Shabtay, I., & Ravid, D. (2010). Cross-linguistic evidence for the nature of age effects in second language acquisition. *Applied Psycholinguistics*, *31*, 413–438. https://doi.org/10.1017/S0142716410000056

Della Putta, P. (2016). The effects of textual enhancement on the acquisition of two non-parallel grammatical features by Spanish-speaking learners of Italian. *Studies in Second Language Acquisition*, *38*, 217–238. https://doi.org/10.1017/S0272263116000073

Dienes, Z., & Scott, R. (2005). Measuring unconscious knowledge: Distinguishing structural knowledge and judgment knowledge. *Psychological Research: An International Journal of Perception, Attention, Memory and Action*, *69*(5–6), 338–351. https://doi.org/10.1007/s00426-004-0208-3

Dörnyei, Z. (2007). *Research methods in applied linguistics*. Oxford: Oxford University Press.

Duffield, N. (2004). Implications of competent gradience. *Moderne Sprachen*, *48*, 95–117.

Duffield, N., Matsuo, A., & Roberts, L. (2007). Acceptable ungrammaticality in sentence matching. *Second Language Research*, *23*, 155–177. https://doi.org/10.1177/0267658307076544

Eckman, F. (1994). Local and long distance anaphora in second—language acquisition. In E. Tarone, S. Gass, & A. Cohen (Eds.), *Research methodology in second—language acquisition* (pp. 207–225). Hillsdale, NJ: Lawrence Erlbaum Associates.

El-Ghazoly, B. (2013). *Feature reassembly and forming syntactic ties: The acquisition of non-canonical agreement in Arabic L2* (Doctoral dissertation). Retrieved from ProQuest. (UMI:3609367).

Elliot, D., Legum, S., & Thompson, S. (1969). Syntactic variation a linguistic data. In R. Binnick et al. (Eds.), *Papers from the fifth regional meeting of the Chicago linguistic society* (pp. 52–59). Chicago: University of Chicago Press, Department of Linguistics.

Ellis, R. (1991). Grammaticality judgments and second language acquisition. *Studies in Second Language Acquisition*, *13*, 161–186. https://doi.org/10.1017/S0272263100009931

Ellis, R. (2004). The definition and measurement of explicit knowledge. *Language Learning*, *54*, 227–275. https://doi.org/10.1111/j.1467-9922.2004.00255.x

Ellis, R. (2005). Measuring implicit and explicit knowledge of a second language: A psychometric study. *Studies in Second Language Acquisition*, *27*, 141–172. https://doi.org/10.1017/S0272263105050096

Ellis, R. (2009a). Introduction. In R. Ellis, S. Loewen, C. Elder, H. Reinders, R. Erlam, & J. Philp (Eds.), *Implicit and explicit knowledge in second language learning, testing and teaching* (pp. 3–25). Bristol, UK: Multilingual Matters.

Ellis, R. (2009b). Measuring implicit and explicit knowledge of a second language. In R. Ellis, S. Loewen, C. Elder, H. Reinders, R. Erlam, & J. Philp (Eds.), *Implicit and explicit knowledge in second language learning, testing and teaching* (pp. 31–64). Bristol, UK: Multilingual Matters.

Ellis, R., & Rathbone, M. (1987). *The acquisition of German in a classroom context.* Mimeograph. London: Ealing College of Higher Education.

Enochson, K., & Culbertson, J. (2015). Collecting psycholinguistic response time data using Amazon Mechanical Turk. *PLoS One, 10.* https://doi.org/10.1371/journal.pone.0116946

Erçetin, G., & Alptekin, C. (2013). The explicit/implicit knowledge distinction and working memory: Implications for second-language reading comprehension. *Applied Psycholinguistics, 34,* 727–753. https://doi.org/10.1017/S0142716411000932

Erlam, R., & Loewen, S. (2010). Implicit ad explicit recasts in L2 oral French interaction. *Canadian Modern Language Review, 66,* 877–905. https://doi.org/10.3138/cmlr.66.6.877

Evanini, K., Higgins, D., & Zechner, K. (2010). *Using Amazon Mechanical Turk for transcription of non-native speech.* Proceedings of the NAACL HLT 2010 Workshop on Creating Speech and Language Data with Amazon's Mechanical Turk (pp. 53–56). Association for Computational Linguistics.

Falk, Y., & Bardel, C. (2011). Object pronouns in German L3 syntax: Evidence for the L2 status factor. *Second Language Research, 27,* 59–82. https://doi.org/10.1177/0267658310386647

Fallah, N., Jabbari, A. A., & Fazilatfar, A. M. (2016). Source(s) of syntactic Cross-Linguistic Influence (CLI): The case of L3 acquisition of English possessives by Mazandarani—Persian bilinguals. *Second Language Research, 32,* 225–245. https://doi.org/10.1177/0267658315618009

Fanselow, G., & Frisch, S. (2006). Effects of processing difficulty on judgments of acceptability. In G. Fanselow, C. Féry, M. Schlesewsky, & R. Vogel (Eds.), *Gradience in grammar* (pp. 291–316). Oxford: Oxford University Press.

Fanselow, G., Schlesewsky, M., Cavar, D., & Kliegl, R. (1999). *Optimal parsing: Syntactic parsing preferences and optimality theory.* Rutgers Optimality Archive, Rutgers State University of New Jersey.

Faretta-Stutenberg, M., & Morgan-Short, K. (2018). Individual differences in context: A neurolinguistic investigation of the role of memory and language use in naturalistic learning contexts. *Second Language Research, 34,* 67–101. doi:10.1177/0267658316684903

Faretta-Stutenberg, M., & Morgan-Short, K. (in press). Contributions of initial proficiency and language use to second language development during study abroad: Behavioral and event-related potential evidence. In C. Sanz & A. Morales Font (Eds.), *Handbook of study abroad research.* London: Routledge.

Featherston, S. (2002). Coreferential objects in German: Experimental evidence on reflexivity. *Linguistische Berichte, 192,* 457–484. Retrieved from www.el.uni-tuebingen.de/sam/papers/ski.paper.pdf

Featherston, S. (2005). That-trace in German. *Lingua, 115,* 1277–1302. https://doi.org/10.1016/j.lingua.2004.04.001

Featherston, S. (2007). Data in generative grammar: The stick and the carrot. *Theoretical Linguistics, 33,* 269–318. https://doi.org/10.1515/TL.2007.020

Featherston, S. (2008). Thermometer judgements as linguistic evidence. In C. Riehl & A. Rothe (Eds.), *Was ist linguistische Evidenz?* (pp. 69–89). Aachen: Shaker Verlag.

Ferreira, F. (2005). Psycholinguistics, formal grammars, and cognitive science. *The Linguistic Review, 22,* 365–380. https://doi.org/10.1515/tlir.2005.22.2-4.365

Follmer, D., Sperling, R., & Suen, H. (2017). The role of MTurk in education research: Advantages, issues, and future directions. *Educational Researcher, 46,* 329–334. https://doi.org/10.3102/0013189X17725519

Forster, K. I., & Dickinson, R. G. (1976). More on the language-as-fixed-effect fallacy: Monte Carlo estimates of error rates for F_1,F_2,F′, and min F′. *Journal of Verbal Learning and Verbal Behavior, 15*, 135–142. https://doi.org/10.1016/0022-5371(76)90014-1

Frick, R. W. (1984). Using both an auditory and a visual short-term store to increase digit span. *Memory and Cognition, 12*, 507–514. https://doi.org/10.3758/BF03198313

Gabriele, A. (2009). Transfer and transition in the SLA of aspect: A bidirectional study of learners of English and Japanese. *Studies in Second Language Acquisition, 31*, 371–402. https://doi.org/10.1017/S0272263109090342

Gass, S. (1979). Language transfer and universal grammatical relations. *Language Learning, 29*, 327–344. https://doi.org/10.1111/j.1467-1770.1979.tb01073.x

Gass, S. (1983). The development of L2 intuitions. *TESOL Quarterly, 17*, 273–291. https://doi.org/10.2307/3586654

Gass, S. (1994). The reliability of second—language grammaticality judgments. In E. Tarone, S. Gass, & A. Cohen (Eds.), *Research methodology in second language acquisition* (pp. 303–322). Hillsdale, NJ: Lawrence Erlbaum Associates.

Gass, S. (2018). Eliciting SLA data: Judgment tasks and elicited imitation. In A. Phakiti, P. De Costa, L. Plonsky, & S. Starfield (Eds.), *Handbook of applied linguistics research methodology* (pp. 313–337). Palgrave Macmillan. https://doi.org/10.1057/978-1-137-59900-1

Gass, S. (in press). Moving forward: Future directions in language learning and teaching. In J. Schweiter & A. Benatti (Eds.), *The Cambridge handbook of language learning*. Cambridge: Cambridge University Press.

Gass, S., & Alvarez Torres, M. (2005). Attention when? An investigation of the ordering effect of input and interaction. *Studies in Second Language Acquisition, 27*, 1–31. https://doi.org/10.1017/S0272263105050011

Gass, S., & Loewen, S., & Plonsky, L. (2018). Coming of age: The past, present, and future of quantitative SLA research. Paper presented at Research Methods Conference, Montpelier, France.

Gass, S., & Mackey, A. (2007). *Data elicitation for second and foreign language research*. Mahwah, NJ: Lawrence Erlbaum Associates.

Gass, S., & Mackey, A. (2015). Input, interaction, and output in second language acquisition. In B. VanPatten & J. Williams (Eds.), *Theories in second language acquisition: An introduction* (pp. 180–206). New York, NY: Routledge.

Gass, S., Mackey, A., Alvarez-Torres, M., & Fernández-García, M. (1999). The effects of task repetition on linguistic output. *Language Learning, 49*, 549–581. https://doi.org/10.1111/0023-8333.00102

Gass, S., & Polio, C. (2014). Methodological influences of "Interlanguage" (1972): Data then and data now. In Z. Han & E. Tarone (Eds.), *Interlanguage: Forty years later* (pp. 147–172). Amsterdam, The Netherlands: John Benjamins.

Gass, S., Svetics, I., & Lemelin, S. (2003). Differential effects of attention. *Language Learning, 53*, 495–543. https://doi.org/ org/10.1111/1467–9922.00233

Geeslin, K. L., & Guijarro-Fuentes, P. (2006). Second language acquisition of variable structures in Spanish by Portuguese speakers. *Language Learning, 56*, 53–107. https://doi.org/10.1111/j.0023-8333.2006.00342.x

Geeslin, K. L., & Guijarro-Fuentes, P. (2008). Variation in contemporary Spanish: Linguistic predictors of estar in four cases of language contact. *Bilingualism: Language and Cognition, 11*, 365–380. https://doi.org/10.1017/S1366728908003593

Gerken, L., & Bever, T. (1986). Linguistic intuitions are the result of interactions between perceptual processes and linguistic universals. *Cognitive Science, 10*, 457–476. https://doi.org/10.1207/s15516709cog1004_3

Gibson, E., & Thomas, J. (1999). Memory limitations and structural forgetting: The perception of complex ungrammatical sentences as grammatical. *Language and Cognitive Processes, 14*, 225–248. https://doi.org/10.1080/016909699386293

Glew, M. (1998). *The acquisition of reflexive pronouns among adult learners of English* (Unpublished doctoral dissertation), Michigan State University, East Lansing, MI.

Godfroid, A., Loewen, S., Jung, S., Park, J. H., Gass, S., & Ellis, R. (2015). Timed and untimed grammaticality judgments measure distinct types of knowledge. *Studies in Second Language Acquisition, 37*, 269–297. https://doi.org/10.1017/S0272263114000850

Gómez-Ruiz, I., Aguilar-Alonso, Á., & Espasa, M. A. (2012). Language impairment in Catalan-Spanish bilinguals with Alzheimer's disease. *Journal of Neurolinguistics, 25*, 552–566. https://doi.org/10.1016/j.jneuroling.2011.06.003

Granena, G. (2014). Language aptitude and long-term achievement in early childhood L2 learners. *Applied linguistics, 35*, 483–503. https://doi.org/10.1093/applin/amu013

Greenbaum, S. (1973). Informant elicitation of data on syntactic variation. *Lingua, 31*, 201–212.

Greenbaum, S. (1977). The linguist as experimenter. In F. Eckman (Eds.), *Current themes in linguistics: Bilingualism, experimental linguistics, and language typologies* (pp. 125–144). New York, NY: Wiley-Blackwell.

Grewendorf, G. (1985). Anaphern bei Objekt-Koreferenz im Deutschen: Ein Problem für die Rektions-Bindungs-Theorie. In W. Abraham (Eds.), *Erklaerende syntax des Deutschen* (pp. 137–171). Tübingen: Narr.

Grewendorf, G. (1988). *Aspekte der deutschen Syntax: Eine Rektions-Bindungs-Analyse*. Tübingen: Narr.

Grey, S., Williams, J. N., & Rebuschat, P. (2014). Incidental exposure and L3 learning of morphosyntax. *Studies in Second Language Acquisition, 36*, 611–645. https://doi.org/10.1017/S0272263113000727

Grey, S., Sanz, C., Morgan-Short, K., & Ullman, M. T. (2018). Bilingual and monolingual adults learning an additional language: ERPs reveal differences in syntactic processing. *Bilingualism: Language and Cognition, 21*, 970–994. https://doi.org/10.1017/S1366728917000426

Guijarro-Fuentes, P., & Larrañaga, M. (2011). Evidence of V to I raising in L2 Spanish. *International Journal of Bilingualism, 15*, 486–520. https://doi.org/10.1177/1367006911425631

Gutiérrez, X. (2012). Implicit knowledge, explicit knowledge, and achievement in second language (L2) Spanish. *Canadian Journal of Applied Linguistics/Revue Canadienne de Linguistique Appliquée, 15*, 20–41. Retrieved from https://journals.lib.unb.ca/index.php/CJAL/article/view/19945/21829

Gutiérrez, X. (2013). The construct validity of grammaticality judgment tests as measures of implicit and explicit knowledge. *Studies in Second Language Acquisition, 35*, 423–449. https://doi.org/10.1017/S0272263113000041

Hahne, A., & Friederici, A. D. (2001). Processing a second language: Late learners' comprehension mechanisms as revealed by event-related brain potentials. *Bilingualism: Language and Cognition, 4*, 123–141. https://doi.org/10.1017/S1366728901000232

Haig, J. (1991). *Universal grammar and second language acquisition: The influence of task type on late learner's access to the subjacency principle*. TESL monograph. Montreal: McGill University.

Han, Y., & Ellis, R. (1998). Implicit knowledge, explicit knowledge and general language proficiency. *Language Teaching Research, 2*, 1–23. https://doi.org/10.1177/136216889800200102

Hartley, J., & Betts, L. R. (2010). Four layouts and a finding: The effects of changes in the order of the verbal labels and numerical values on Likert-type scales. *International Journal of Social Research Methodology*, *13*, 17–27. https://doi.org/10.1080/13645570802648077

Hartshorne, J., Tenenbaum, J., & Pinker, S. (in press). A critical period for second language acquisition: Evidence from 2/3 million English speakers. *Cognition*. https://doi.org/org/10.1016/j.cognition.2018.04.007

Hawkins, R. (1987). Markedness and the acquisition of the English dative alternation by L2 speakers. *Second Language Research*, *3*, 20–55. doi:10.1177/026765838700300104

Hedgcock, J. (1993). Well-formed vs. ill-formed strings in L2 metalingual tasks: Specifying features of grammaticality judgements. *Second Language Research*, *9*, 1–21. https://doi.org/10.1177/026765839300900101

Hill, A. (1961). Grammaticality. *Word*, *17*, 1–10.

Hofmeister, P., Culicover, P., & Winkler, S. (2015). Effects of processing on the acceptability of "frozen" extraposed constituents. *Syntax-a Journal of Theoretical Experimental and Interdisciplinary Research*, *18*, 464–483. https://doi.org/org/10.1111/synt.12036

Hofmeister, P., Jaeger, T., Arnon, I., Sag, I., & Snider, N. (2013). The source ambiguity problem: Distinguishing the effects of grammar and processing on acceptability judgment. *Language and Cognitive Processes*, *28*, 48–87. https://doi.org/10.1080/01690965.2011.572401

Hofmeister, P., Staum, C. L., & Sag, I. (2012). How do individual cognitive differences relate to acceptability judgments? A reply to Sprouse, Wagers, and Philipps. *Language*, *88*, 390–400. https://doi.org/10.1353/lan.2012.0025

Hopp, H. (2009). The syntax-discourse interface in near-native L2 acquisition: Off-line and on-line performance. *Bilingualism: Language and Cognition*, *12*, 463–483. https://doi.org/10.1017/S1366728909990253

Hopp, H. (2010). Ultimate attainment in L2 inflection: Performance similarities between non-native and native speakers. *Lingua*, *120*, 901–931. https://doi.org/10.1016/j.lingua.2009.06.004

Householder, F. (1973). On arguments from asterisks. *Foundations of Language*, *10*, 365–376.

Hu, G. (2002). Psychological constraints on the utility of metalinguistic knowledge in second language production. *Studies in Second Language Acquisition*, *24*, 347–386. https://doi.org/10.1017/S0272263102003017

Huang, B. H. (2014). The effects of age on second language grammar and speech production. *Journal of Psycholinguistic Research*, *43*, 397–420. https://doi.org/10.1007/s10936-013-9261-7

Hulk, A. (1991). Parameter setting and the acquisition of word order in L2 French. *Second Language Research*, 7, 1–34. https://doi.org/10.1177/026765839100700101

Hwang, S., & Lardiere, D. (2013). Plural-marking in L2 Korean: A feature-based approach. *Second Language Research*, *29*, 57–86. https://doi.org/10.1177/0267658312461496

Hyltenstam, K. (1977). Implicational patterns in interlanguage syntax variation. *Language Learning*, *27*, 383–410. https://doi.org/10.1111/j.1467-1770.1977.tb00129.x

Inagaki, S. (2001). Motion verbs with goal PPs in the L2 acquisition of English and Japanese. *Studies in Second Language Acquisition*, *23*, 153–170. https://doi.org/10.1017/S0272263101002029

Indrarathne, B., & Kormos, J. (2017). Attentional processing of input in explicit and implicit conditions. *Studies in Second Language Acquisition*, *39*, 401–430. https://doi.org/10.1017/S027226311600019X

Ionin, T. (2012). Formal theory-based methodologies. In A. Mackey & S. Gass (Eds.), *Research methods in second language acquisition: A practical guide* (pp. 30–52). Oxford: Wiley-Blackwell.

Ionin, T., & Montrul, S. (2009). Article use and generic reference: Parallels between L1-and L2-acquisition. In M. del Pilar, G. Mayo, & R. Hawkins (Eds.), *Second language acquisition of articles: Empirical findings and theoretical implications* (pp. 147–173). Amsterdam, The Netherlands: John Benjamins.

Ionin, T., & Montrul, S. (2010). The role of L1 transfer in the interpretation of articles with definite plurals in L2 English. *Language Learning, 60*, 877–925. https://doi.org/10.1111/j.1467-9922.2010.00577.x

Ionin, T., & Zyzik, E. (2014). Judgment and interpretation tasks in second language research. *Annual Review of Applied Linguistics, 34*, 37–64. https://doi.org/10.1017/S0267190514000026

Izumi, S., Bigelow, M., Fujiwara, M., & Fearnow, S. (1999). Testing the output hypothesis: Effects of Output on Noticing and second language acquisition. *Studies in Second Language Acquisition, 21*, 421–452. https://doi.org/10.1017/S0272263199003034

Jegerski, J., & VanPatten, B. (2014). *Research methods in second language psycholinguistics*. New York, NY: Routledge.

Jiang, N. (2012). *Conducting reaction time research in second language studies*. New York, NY: Routledge.

Johnson, J. S. (1992). Critical period effects in second language acquisition: The effect of written versus auditory materials on the assessment of grammatical competence. *Language Learning, 42*, 217–248. https://doi.org/10.1111/j.1467-1770.1992.tb00708.x

Johnson, J. S., & Newport, E. (1989). Critical period effects in second language learning: The influence of maturational state on the acquisition of English as a second language. *Cognitive Psychology, 21*, 60–99. https://doi.org/10.1016/0010-0285(89)90003-0

Johnson, J. S., & Newport, E. (1991). Critical period effects on universal properties of language: The status of subjacency in the acquisition of a second language. *Cognition, 39*, 215–258. https://doi.org/10.1016/0010-0277(91)90054-8

Juffs, A. (2001). Discussion: Verb classes, event structure, and second language learners' knowledge of semantics—syntax correspondences. *Studies in Second Language Acquisition, 23*, 305–314. https://doi.org/10.1017/S027226310100208X

Juffs, A., & Harrington, M. (1996). Garden path sentences and error data in second language sentence processing. *Language Learning, 46*, 283–323. https://doi.org/10.1111/j.1467-1770.1996.tb01237.x

Juffs, A., & Rodríguez, G. (2008). Some notes on working memory in college-educated and low-educated learners of English as a second language in the United States. In M. Young-Scholten (Eds.), *Low-educated second language and literacy acquisition: Research, policy and practice* (Vol. 3, pp. 33–48). Newcastle-Upon-Tyne, Durham: Rounduit.

Kellerman, E. (1985). If at first you *do* succeed. In S. Gass & C. Madden (Eds.), *Input in second language acquisition* (pp. 345–353). Rowley, MA: Newbury House.

Kellerman, E. (1987). *Aspects of transferability in second language acquisition* (Unpublished doctoral dissertation), Katholieke Universiteit te Nijmegen, Nijmegen.

Khatib, M., & Nikouee, M. (2012). Planned focus on form: Automatization of procedural knowledge. *RELC Journal, 43*, 187–201. https://doi.org/10.1177/0033688212450497

Knightley, L., Jun, S-A., Oh, J., & Au, T. (2003). Production benefits of childhood overhearing. *The Journal of the Acoustical Society of America, 114*, 465-474. https://doi.org/10.1121/1.1577560

Knowlton, B. J., & Moody, T. D. (2008). Procedural learning in humans. In J. H. Bryne (Ed.), *Learning and memory: A comprehensive reference*: Vol. 3. *Memory systems* (pp. 321–340). Oxford: Academic Press, Elsevier.

Koerner, E. F. K. (1996/1997). Notes on the history of the concept of language as a system 'Où tout se tient'. *Linguistica Atlantica, 19*, 1–20.

Kraš, T. (2011). Acquiring the syntactic constraints on auxiliary change under restructuring in L2 Italian. *Linguistic Approaches to Bilingualism, 1*, 413–438. https://doi.org/10.1075/lab.1.4.03kra

Krashen, S. (1982). *Principles and practice in second language acquisition*. London: Pergamon.

Kuperman, V., Stadthagen-Gonzalez, H., & Brysbaert, M. (2012). Age-of-acquisition ratings for 30,000 English words. *Behavioral Research, 44*, 978–990. https://doi.org/10.3758/s13428-012-0209-x

Kupisch, T. (2012). Specific and generic subjects in the Italian of German-Italian simultaneous bilinguals and L2 learners. *Bilingualism: Language and Cognition, 15*, 736–756. https://doi.org/10.1017/S1366728911000691

Kweon, S-O., & Bley-Vroman, R. (2011). Acquisition of the constraints on "wanna" contraction by advanced second language learners: Universal grammar and imperfect knowledge. *Second Language Research, 27*, 207–228. https://doi.org/10.1177/0267658310375756

Labov, W. (1975). Empirical foundations of linguistic theory. In R. Austerlitz (Eds.), *Papers of the first Golden Anniversary Symposium of the Linguistic Society of America, held at the University of Massachusetts, Amherst, on July 24 and 25, 1974* (pp. 77–133). Lisse: Peter de Ridder.

Labov, W. (1996). When intuitions fail. In L. McNair, K. Singer, L. Dobrin, & M. Aucoin (Eds.), *Papers from the parasession on theory and data in linguistics (Volume 32)* (pp. 77–106). Chicago: Chicago Linguistic Society.

Lakoff, G. (1973). Fuzzy grammar and the performance/ competence terminology game. In C. Corum, T. Smith-Stark, & A. Weiser (Eds.), *Papers from the ninth regional meeting* (pp. 271–291). Chicago: Chicago Linguistic Society.

Lakshmanan, U., & Teranishi, K. (1994). Preferences versus grammaticality judgments: Some methodological issues concerning the governing category parameter in second language acquisition. In E. Tarone, S. Gass, & A. Cohen (Eds.), *Research methodology in second language acquisition* (pp. 185–206). Hillsdale, NJ: Lawrence Erlbaum Associates.

Lantolf, J. P., Thorne, S. L., & Poehner, M. E. (2015). Sociocultural theory and second language development. In B. VanPatten & J. Williams (Eds.), *Theories in second language acquisition: An introduction* (pp. 207–226). New York, NY: Routledge.

Lardiere, D. (2008). Feature assembly in second language acquisition. In J. M. Liceras, H. Zobl, & H. Goodluck (Eds.), *The role of formal features in second language acquisition* (pp. 106–140). New York, NY: Lawrence Erlbaum Associates.

Lardiere, D. (2009). Some thoughts on the contrastive analysis of features in second language acquisition. *Second Language Research, 25*, 173–227. https://doi.org/10.1177/0267658308100283

Larson-Hall, J. (2008). Weighing the benefits of studying a foreign language at a younger starting age in a minimal input situation. *Second Language Research, 24*, 35–63. https://doi.org/10.1177/0267658307082981

Larson-Hall, J. (2016). *A guide to doing statistics in second language research using SPSS and R*. New York, NY: Routledge.

Larson-Hall, J., & Herrington, R. (2009). Improving data analysis in second language acquisition by utilizing modern developments in applied statistics. *Applied Linguistics, 31*, 368–390. https://doi.org/10.1093/applin/amp038

Lenneberg, E. (1967). *Biological foundations of language*. New York, NY: Wiley-Blackwell.

Leow, R. (1996). Grammaticality judgment tasks and second-language development. In J. E. Alatis, C. A. Straehle, M. Ronkin, & B. Gallenberger (Eds.), *Georgetown University round table on languages and linguistics* (pp. 126–139). Washington, DC: Georgetown University Press.

Levelt, W., van Gent, J., Haans, A., & Meijers, A. (1977). Grammaticality, paraphrase and imagery. In S. Greenbaum (Eds.), *Acceptability in language* (pp. 87–101). The Hague: Mouton.

Li, S. (2012). The effect of input-based practice on pragmatic development of requests in L2 Chinese. *Language Learning, 62*, 403–438. https://doi.org/10.1111/j.1467-9922.2011.00629.x

Li, S. (2013). The interactions between the effects of implicit and explicit feedback and individual differences in language analytic ability and working memory. *The Modern Language Journal, 97*, 634–654. https://doi.org/10.1111/j.1540-4781.2013.12030.x

Li, S., Ellis, R., & Zhu, Y. (2016). Task-based versus task-supported language instruction: An experimental study. *Annual Review of Applied Linguistics, 36*, 205–229. https://doi.org/10.1017/S0267190515000069

Liceras, J. (1983). *Markedness, contrastive analysis and the acquisition of Spanish syntax by English speakers* (Unpublished doctoral thesis), University of Toronto, Toronto.

Linacre, J. M. (1988). *LinacreFacets Rasch analysis computer program*. Chicago: MESA Press.

Loewen, S. (2009). Grammaticality judgment tests and the measurement of implicit and explicit L2 knowledge. In R. Ellis, S. Loewen, C. Elder, H. Reinders, R. Erlam, & J. Philp (Eds.), *Implicit and explicit knowledge in second language learning, testing and teaching* (pp. 94–112). Bristol, UK: Multilingual Matters.

Loewen, S. (2015). *Introduction to instructed second language acquisition*. New York, NY: Routledge.

Long, M. H. (1996). The role of the linguistic environment in second language acquisition. In W. C. Ritchie & T. K. Bhatia (Eds.), *Handbook of language acquisition: Second language acquisition* (pp. 413–468). New York, NY: Academic Press.

Lozano, C. (2002). Knowledge of expletive and pronominal subjects by learners of Spanish. *ITL International Journal of Applied Linguistics, 135–136*, 37–60.

Mackey, A., Adams, R., Stafford, C., & Winke, P. (2010). Exploring the relationship between modified output and working memory capacity. *Language Learning, 60*, 501–533. https://doi.org/10.1111/j.1467-9922.2010.00565.x

Mackey, A., & Gass., S. (2016). *Second language research: Methodology and design*. New York, NY: Routledge.

Macmillan, N. A., & Creelman, C. D. (2004). *Detection theory: A user's guide*. New York: Psychology Press.

Mai, Z., & Yuan, B. (2016). Uneven reassembly of tense, telicity and discourse features in L2 acquisition of the Chinese shi . . . de cleft construction. *Second Language Research, 32*, 247–276. doi:10.1177/0267658315623323

Marantz, A. (2005). Generative linguistics within the cognitive neuroscience of language. *The Linguistic Review, 22*, 429–445. https://doi.org/10.1515/tlir.2005.22.2-4.429

Marsden, E. (2006). Exploring input processing in the classroom: An experimental comparison of processing instruction and enriched input. *Language Learning, 56*, 507–566. https://doi.org/10.1111/j.1467-9922.2006.00375.x

Marsden, H. (2008). Pair-list readings in Korean-Japanese, Chinese-Japanese and English-Japanese interlanguage. *Second Language Research, 24*, 189–226. https://doi.org/10.1177/0267658307086301

Marsden, E., & Chen, H-Y. (2011). The roles of structured input activities in processing instruction and the kinds of knowledge they promote. *Language Learning, 61*, 1058–1098. https://doi.org/10.1111/j.1467-9922.2011.00661.x

Marsden, E., Mackey, A., & Plonsky, L. (2016). The IRIS Repository: Advancing research practice and methodology. In A. Mackey & E. Marsden (Eds.), *Advancing methodology and practice: The IRIS repository of instruments for research into second languages* (pp. 1–21). New York, NY: Routledge.

McDaniel, D., McKee, C., & Cairns, H. S. (1996). *Methods for assessing children's syntax*. Cambridge, MA: MIT Press.

McDonald, J. (2008). Grammaticality judgments in children: The role of age, working memory and phonological ability. *Journal of Child Language, 35*, 247–268. https://doi.org/10.1017/S0305000907008367

McManus, K., & Marsden, E. (2017). L1 explicit instruction can improve L2 online and offline performance. *Studies in Second Language Acquisition, 39*, 459–492. https://doi.org/10.1017/S027226311600022X

Meara, P. (2005). *LLAMA language aptitude tests*. Swansea: Lognostics.

Meulman, N., Wieling, M., Sprenger, S. A., Stowe, L. A., & Schmid, M. S. (2015). Age effects in L2 grammar processing as revealed by ERPs and how (not) to study them. *PLoS One, 10*. https://doi.org/10.1371/journal.pone.0143328

Miller, A. K. (2015). Intermediate traces and intermediate learners. *Studies in Second Language Acquisition, 37*, 487–516. https://doi.org/10.1017/S0272263114000588

Miller, A. K., Leonard, L., & Finneran, D. (2008). Grammaticality judgments in adolescents with and without language impairment. *Journal of Language Communication Disorders, 43*, 346–360. https://doi.org/10.1080/13682820701546813

Mills, J., & Hemsley, G. (1976). The effect of level of education on judgments of grammatical acceptability. *Language and Speech, 19*, 324–342. https://doi.org/10.1177/002383097601900404

Montrul, S. (1999). Causative errors with unaccusative verbs in L2 Spanish. *Second Language Research, 15*, 191–219. https://doi.org/10.1191/026765899669832752

Montrul, S., & Bowles, M. (2009). Back to basics: Incomplete knowledge of differential object marking in Spanish heritage speakers. *Bilingualism: Language and Cognition, 12*, 363–383. https://doi.org/10.1017/S1366728909990071

Montrul, S., Davidson, J., De La Fuente, I., & Foote, R. (2014). Early language experience facilitates the processing of gender agreement in Spanish heritage speakers. *Bilingualism: Language and Cognition, 17*, 118–138. https://doi.org/10.1017/S1366728913000114

Montrul, S., Dias, R., & Santos, H. (2011). Clitics and object expression in the L3 acquisition of Brazilian Portuguese: Structural similarity matters for transfer. *Second Language Research, 27*, 21–58. https://doi.org/10.1177/0267658310386649

Morgan-Short, K., Faretta-Stutenberg, M., Brill-Schuetz, K. A., Carpenter, H., & Wong, P. C. (2014). Declarative and procedural memory as individual differences in second language acquisition. *Bilingualism: Language and Cognition, 17*, 56–72. https://doi.org/10.1017/S1366728912000715

Morgan-Short, K., Sanz, C., Steinhauer, K., & Ullman, M. T. (2010). Second language acquisition of gender agreement in explicit and implicit training conditions: An event-related potential study. *Language Learning, 60*, 154–193. https://doi.org/10.1111/j.1467-9922.2009.00554.x

Mueller, J. L., Girgsdies, S., & Friederici, A. D. (2008). The impact of semantic-free second-language training on ERPs during case processing. *Neuroscience letters, 443*, 77–81. https://doi.org/10.1016/j.neulet.2008.07.054

Muñoz, C., & Singleton, D. (2011). A critical review of age-related research on L2 ultimate attainment. *Language Teaching, 44*, 1–35. https://doi.org/10.1017/S0261444810000327

Murphy, V. A. (1997). The effect of modality on a grammaticality judgement task. *Second Language Research, 13*, 34–65. https://doi.org/10.1191/026765897671676818

Myers, J. (2009a). Syntactic judgment experiments. *Language and Linguistics Compass, 3*, 406–423. https://doi.org/10.1111/j.1749-818x.2008.00113.x

Myers, J. (2009b). The design and analysis of small-scale syntactic judgment experiments *Lingua, 119*, 425–444. https://doi.org/10.1016/j.lingua.2008.09.003

Nabei, T., & Swain, M. (2002). Learner awareness of recasts in classroom interaction: A case study of an adult EFL student's second language learning. *Language Awareness, 11*, 43–63. https://doi.org/10.1080/09658410208667045

Nagano, T. (2015). Acquisition of English verb transitivity by native speakers of Japanese. *Linguistic Approaches to Bilingualism, 5*, 322–355. https://doi.org/10.1075/lab.5.3.02nag

Nagata, H. (1991). On-line judgments of grammaticality of sentences involving rule violations. *Psychologia: An International Journal of Psychology in the Orient, 34*, 171–176.

Negri, M., & Mehdad, Y. (2010). *Creating a bi-lingual entailment corpus through translations with Mechanical Turk: $100 for a 10-day rush*. Proceedings of the NAACL HLT 2010 Workshop on Creating Speech and Language Data with Amazon's Mechanical Turk (pp. 212–216). Association for Computational Linguistics.

Neubauer, K., & Clahsen, H. (2009). Decomposition of inflected words in a second language: An experimental study of German participles. *Studies in Second Language Acquisition, 31*, 403–435. https://doi.org/10.1017/S0272263109090354

Newmeyer, F. (2007). Commentary on Sam Featherston, 'Data in generative grammar: The stick and the carrot'. *Theoretical Linguistics, 33*, 395–399. https://doi.org/10.1515/TL.2007.026

Norouzian, R., & Plonsky, L. (2018). Eta- and partial eta-squared in L2 research: A cautionary review and guide to more appropriate usage. *Second Language Research, 34*, 257–271. https://doi.org/10.1177/0267658316684904

Oh, E. (2010). Recovery from first-language transfer: The second language acquisition of English double objects by Korean speakers. *Second Language Research, 26*, 407–439. https://doi.org/10.1177/0267658310365786

Pae, H. K., Schanding, B., Kwon, Y. J., & Lee, Y. W. (2014). Animacy effect and language specificity: Judgment of unaccusative verbs by Korean learners of English as a foreign language. *Journal of Psycholinguistic Research, 43*, 187–207. https://doi.org/10.1007/s10936-013-9246-6

Paradis, M. (2011). Principles underlying the Bilingual Aphasia Test (BAT) and its uses. *Clinical Linguistics & Phonetics, 25*, 427–443. https://doi.org/10.3109/02699206.2011.560326

Parodi, T., & Tsimpli, I-M. (2005). "Real" and apparent optionality in second language grammars: Finiteness and pronouns in null operator structures. *Second Language Research, 21*, 250–285. https://doi.org/10.1191/0267658305sr248oa

Perek, F., & Goldberg, A. E. (2017). Linguistic generalization on the basis of function and constraints on the basis of statistical preemption. *Cognition, 168*, 276–293. https://doi.org/org/10.1016/j.cognition.2017.06.019

Perpiñán, S. (2015). L2 grammar and L2 processing in the acquisition of Spanish prepositional relative clauses. *Bilingualism: Language and Cognition, 18*, 577–596. https://doi.org/10.1017/S1366728914000583

Phakiti, A. (2014). Experimental research methods in language learning. London: Bloomsbury.

Philp, J., & Iwashita, N. (2013). Talking, tuning in and noticing: Exploring the benefits of output in task-based peer interaction. *Language Awareness*, *22*, 353–370. https://doi.org/10.1080/09658416.2012.758128

Pienemann, M. (1998). *Language processing and second language development: Processability theory*. Amsterdam, The Netherlands: John Benjamins.

Pienemann, M. (2005). Discussing PT. In M. Pienemann (Ed.), *Cross-linguistic aspects of processability theory* (pp. 61–83). Amsterdam, The Netherlands: John Benjamins.

Plonsky, L. (2012). Replication, meta-analysis, and generalizability. In G. Porte (Eds.), *Replication research in applied linguistics* (pp. 116–132). New York, NY: Cambridge University Press.

Plonsky, L., & Derrick, D. J. (2016). A meta-analysis of reliability coefficients in second language research. *The Modern Language Journal*, *100*, 538–553. https://doi.org/10.1111/modl.12335

Plonsky, L., & Ghanbar, H. (2018). Multiple regression in L2 research: A methodological synthesis and guide to interpreting R^2 values. *The Modern Language Journal*, *102*, 713–731.

Plonsky, L., Marsden, E., Crowther, D., Gass, S., & Spinner, P. (in press). A methodological synthesis of judgment tasks in second language research. *Second Language Research*.

Plonsky, L., & Oswald, F. L. (2014). How big is 'big'? Interpreting effect sizes in L2 research. *Language Learning*, *64*, 878–912. https://doi.org/10.1111/lang.12079

Prentza, A. (2014). *Pronominal subjects in English L2 acquisition and in L1 Greek: Issues of interpretation, use and L1 transfer*. Major Trends in Theoretical and Applied Linguistics 2: Selected Papers from the 20th ISTAL, 2, 369.

Purpura, J. (2004). *Assessing grammar*. Cambridge: Cambridge University Press.

Quene, H., & van den Bergh, H. (2004). On multi-level modelling of data from repeated measures designs: A tutorial. *Speech Communication*, *43*, 103–121. https://doi.org/10.1016/j.specom.2004.02.004

Quene, H., & van den Bergh, H. (2008). Examples of mixed-effects modelling with crossed random effects and with binomial data. *Journal of Memory and Language*, *59*, 413–425. https://doi.org/10.1016/j.jml.2008.02.002

Rebuschat, P. (2013). Measuring implicit and explicit knowledge in second language research. *Language Learning*, *63*, 595–626. https://doi.org/10.1111/lang.12010

Rebuschat, P., & Williams, J. N. (2012). Implicit and explicit knowledge in second language acquisition. *Applied Psycholinguistics*, *33*, 829–856. https://doi.org/ 10.1017/S0142716411000580

Reis, A., & Castro-Caldas, A. (1997). Illiteracy: A cause for biased cognitive development. *Journal of the International Neuropsychological Society*, *3*, 444–450. Retrieved from www.ncbi.nlm.nih.gov/pubmed/9322403

Richardson, J. (2011). Eta squared and partial eta squared as measures of effect size in education research. *Educational Research Review*, *6*, 135–147. https://doi.org/10.1016/j.edurev.2010.12.001

Ritchie, W. C. (1974). *On the perceptual nature of island constraints: Evidence from an adult-acquired language*. Paper delivered at 1974 LSA annual meeting, New York, NY.

Ritchie, W. C. (1978). The right roof constraint in adult-acquired language. In W. C. Ritchie (Ed.), *Second language acquisition research: Issues and implications*. New York: Academic Press.

Robenalt, C., & Goldberg, A. E. (2015). Judgment evidence for statistical preemption: It is relatively better to vanish than to disappear a rabbit, but a lifeguard can equally well backstroke or swim children to shore. *Cognitive Linguistics*, *26*, 467–503. https://doi.org/10.1515/cog-2015-0004

Robenalt, C., & Goldberg, A. E. (2016). Nonnative speakers do not take competing alternative expressions into account the way native speakers do. *Language Learning, 66*, 60–93. https://doi.org/10.1111/lang.12149

Roberts, L., & Liszka, S. (2013). Processing tense/aspect agreement violations online in the second language: A self-paced reading study with French and German L2 learners of English. *Second Language Research, 29*, 413–439. https://doi.org/10.1177/0267658313503171

Rodríguez Silva, L., & Roehr-Brackin, K. (2016). Perceived learning difficulty and actual performance: Explicit and implicit knowledge of L2 English grammar points among instructed adult learners. *Studies in Second Language Acquisition, 38*, 317–340. https://doi.org/10.1017/S0272263115000340

Ross, J. (1972). The category squish: Edstation Hauptwort. In P. Peranteau, J. Lei, & G. Phares (Eds.), *Papers from the eighth regional meeting* (pp. 316–338). Chicago: Chicago Linguistic Society.

Rosselli, M., Ardila, A., & Rosas, P. (1990). Neuropsychological assessment in illiterates: II. Language and praxic abilities. *Brain and Cognition, 12*, 281–296. https://doi.org/10.1016/0278-2626(90)90020-O

Rothman, J., & Iverson, M. (2013). Islands and objects in L2 Spanish: Do you know the learners who drop? *Studies in Second Language Acquisition, 35*, 589–618. https://doi.org/10.1017/S0272263113000387

Sabourin, L., Stowe, L. A., & de Haan, G. J. (2006). Transfer effects in learning a second language grammatical gender system. *Second Language Research, 22*, 1–29. https://doi.org/10.1191/0267658306sr259oa

Sagarra, N., & Herschensohn, J. (2011). Proficiency and animacy effects on L2 gender agreement processes during comprehension. *Language Learning, 61*, 80–116. https://doi.org/10.1111/j.1467-9922.2010.00588.x

Schachter, J. (1989). A new look at an old classic. *Second Language Research, 5*, 30–42. https://doi.org/10.1177/026765838900500102

Schachter, J., Tyson, A. F., & Diffley, F. J. (1976). Learner intuitions of grammaticality. *Language Learning, 26*, 67–76. https://doi.org/10.1111/j.1467-1770.1976.tb00260.x

Schmidt, R., & McCreary, C. (1977). Standard and super-standard English: Recognition and use of prescriptive rules by native and non-native speakers. *TESOL Quarterly, 11*, 415–429.

Schulz, B. (2011). Syntactic creativity in second language English: "Wh"-scope marking in Japanese-English interlanguage. *Second Language Research, 27*, 313–341. https://doi.org/10.1177/0267658310390503

Schütze, C. (1996). *The empirical base of linguistics: Grammaticality judgments and linguistic methodology*. Chicago: University of Chicago Press.

Schütze, C., & Sprouse, J. (2013). Judgment data. In R. Podesva & D. Sharma (Eds.), *Research methods in linguistics* (pp. 27–50). Cambridge: Cambridge University Press.

Selinker, L. (1972). Interlanguage. *International Review of Applied Linguistics in Language Teaching, 10*, 209–232. https://doi.org/10.1515/iral.1972.10.1-4.209

Singleton, D. (2001). Age and second language acquisition. *Annual Review of Applied Linguistics, 21*, 77–89. https://doi.org/10.1017/S0267190501000058

Slavoff, G. R., & Johnson, J. S. (1995). The effects of age on the rate of learning a second language. *Studies in Second Language Acquisition, 17*, 1–16. https://doi.org/10.1017/S0272263100013723

Smith, M. (2016). L2 learners and the apparent problem of morphology: Evidence from L2 Japanese. In A. Benati & S. Yamashita (Eds.), *Theory, research, and pedagogy in learning and teaching Japanese*. London: Palgrave Macmillan. https://doi.org/10.1057/978-1-137-49892-2_5

Smith, N. (2000). Foreword to *New horizons in the study of language and mind*. Ed. N. Chomsky. Cambridge: Cambridge University Press.

Soler, I. G. (2015). The logical problem of second language acquisition of argument structure: Recognizing aspectual distinctions in Spanish psych-predicates. *International Journal of Bilingualism, 19*, 627–645. https://doi.org/10.1177/1367006914527185

Sorace, A. (1992). *Lexical conditions on syntactic knowledge: Auxiliary selection in native and non-native grammars of Italian* (Ph.D. dissertation), University of Edinburgh, Edinburgh.

Sorace, A. (2010). Using magnitude estimation in developmental linguistic research. In E. Blom & S. Unsworth (Eds.), *Experimental methods in language acquisition research* (pp. 57–72). Amsterdam, The Netherlands: John Benjamins.

Sorace, A., & Keller, F. (2005). Gradience in linguistic data. *Lingua, 115*, 1497–1524. https://doi.org/10.1016/j.lingua.2004.07.002

Spada, N., & Lightbown, P. M. (1999). Instruction, first language influence, and developmental readiness in second language acquisition. *The Modern Language Journal, 83*, 1–22. https://doi.org/10.1111/0026-7902.00002

Spada, N., Shiu, J. L-J., & Tomita, Y. (2015). Validating an elicited imitation task as a measure of implicit knowledge: Comparisons with other validation studies. *Language Learning, 65*, 723–751. https://doi.org/10.1111/lang.12129

Spencer, N. (1973). Differences between linguists and nonlinguists in intuitions of grammaticality-acceptability. *Journal of Psycholinguistic Research, 2*, 83–98. https://doi.org/10.1007/BF01067203

Spinner, P. (2013). Language production and reception: A processability theory study. *Language Learning, 63*, 704–739. https://doi.org/10.1111/lang.12022

Sprouse, J. (2008). The differential sensitivity of acceptability judgments to processing effects. *Linguistic Inquiry, 39*, 686–694. https://doi.org/10.1162/ling.2008.39.4.686

Sprouse, J. (2011a). A test of the cognitive assumptions of magnitude estimation: Commutativity does not hold for acceptability judgments. *Language, 87*, 274–289. https://doi.org/www.jstor.org/stable/23011625

Sprouse, J. (2011b). A validation of Amazon mechanical Turk for the collection of acceptability judgments in linguistic theory. *Behavior Research Methods, 43*, 155–167. https://doi.org/10.3758/s13428-010-0039-7

Sprouse, J. (2013). Acceptability judgments. *Oxford Bibliographies Online: Linguistics*. https://doi.org/10.1093/OBO/9780199772810-0097

Sprouse, J., & Almeida, D. (2012). Assessing the reliability of textbook data in syntax: Adger's core syntax. *Journal of Linguistics, 48*, 609–652. https://doi.org/10.1017/S0022226712000011

Sprouse, J., & Almeida, D. (2017a). Setting the empirical record straight: Acceptability judgments appear to be reliable, robust, and replicable. *Behavioral and Brain Sciences, 40*, E311. doi:10.1017/S0140525X17000590

Sprouse, J., & Almeida, D. (2017b). Design sensitivity and statistical power in acceptability judgment experiments. *Glossa: A Journal of General Linguistics, 2, 14*. https://doi.org/10.5334/gjgl.236

Sprouse, J., Schütze, C., & Almeida, D. (2013). A comparison of informal and formal acceptability judgments using a random sample from Linguistic Inquiry 2001–2010. *Lingua, 134*, 219–248. https://doi.org/10.1016/j.lingua.2013.07.002

Sprouse, J., Wagers, M., & Phillips, C. (2012). A test of the relation between working memory capacity and island effects. *Language, 88*, 82–123. https://doi.org/10.1353/lan.2012.0004

Stafford, C. A. (2011). Bilingualism and enhanced attention in early adulthood. *International Journal of Bilingual Education and Bilingualism, 14*, 1–22. https://doi.org/10.1080/13670050903568209

Stafford, C. A. (2013). What's on your mind? How private speech mediates cognition during initial non-primary language learning. *Applied linguistics, 34*, 151–172. https://doi.org/10.1093/applin/ams039

Stevens, S. (1956). The direct estimation of sensory magnitudes: Loudness. *The American Journal of Psychology, 69*, 1–25.

Stevens, S. (1975). *Psychophysics: Introduction to its perceptual, neural, and social prospects.* New York, NY: John Wiley.

Stringer, D., Burghardt, B., Seo, H-K., & Wang, Y-T. (2011). Straight on through to Universal Grammar: Spatial modifiers in second language acquisition. *Second Language Research, 27*, 289–311. https://doi.org/10.1177/0267658310384567

Suzuki, Y., & DeKeyser, R. M. (2015). Comparing elicited imitation and word monitoring as measures of implicit knowledge. *Language Learning, 65*, 860–895. https://doi.org/10.1111/lang.12138

Suzuki, Y. & DeKeyser, R. (2017). The interface of explicit and implicit knowledge in a second language: Insights from individual differences in cognitive aptitudes. *Language Learning, 67*, 747–790.

Tagarelli, K., Ruiz, S., Vega, J., & Rebuschat, P. (2016). Variability in second language learning: The roles of individual differences, learning conditions, and linguistic complexity. *Studies in Second Language Acquisition, 38*, 293–316. https://doi.org/10.1017/S0272263116000036

Takimoto, M. (2008). The effects of deductive and inductive instruction on the development of language learners' pragmatic competence. *The Modern Language Journal, 92*, 369 386. https://doi.org/10.1111/j.1540-4781.2008.00752.x

Thomas, M. (1989). The interpretation of English reflexive pronouns by non—native speakers. *Studies in Second Language Acquisition, 11*, 281–303. https://doi.org/10.1017/S0272263100008147

Thomas, M. (1991). Universal Grammar and the interpretation of reflexives in a second language. *Language, 67*, 211–239. https://doi.org/10.1353/lan.1991.0065

Thomas, M. (1993). *Knowledge of reflexives in a second language.* Amsterdam, The Netherlands and Philadelphia: John Benjamins.

Thomas, M. (1994). Assessment of L2 proficiency in second language acquisition research. *Language Learning, 44*, 307–336. https://doi.org/10.1111/j.1467-1770.1994.tb01104.x

Thomas, M. (1995). Acquisition of the Japanese reflexive zibun and movement of anaphors in logical form. *Second Language Research, 11*, 206–234. https://doi.org/10.1177/026765839501100302

Tolentino, L. C., & Tokowicz, N. (2014). Cross-language similarity modulates effectiveness of second language grammar instruction. *Language Learning, 64*, 279–309. https://doi.org/10.1111/lang.12048

Toth, P. D. (2006). Processing instruction and a role for output in second language acquisition. *Language Learning, 56*, 319–385. https://doi.org/10.1111/j.0023-8333.2006.00349.x

Toth, P. D. (2008). Teacher- and learner-led discourse in task-based grammar instruction: Providing procedural assistance for L2 morphosyntactic development. *Language Learning, 58*, 237–283. https://doi.org/10.1111/j.1467-9922.2008.00441.x

Toth, P. D., & Guijarro-Fuentes, P. (2013). The impact of instruction on second language implicit knowledge: Evidence against encapsulation. *Applied Psycholinguistics, 34*, 1163–1193. https://doi.org/10.1017/S0142716412000197

Trahey, M. (1996). Positive evidence in second language acquisition: Some long-term effects. *Second Language Research, 12*, 111–139. doi:10.1177/026765839601200201

Trahey, M., & White, L. (1993). Positive evidence and preemption in the second language classroom. *Studies in Second Language Acquisition, 15*, 181–204. https://doi.org/10.1017/S0272263100011955

Tremblay, A. (2005). Theoretical and methodological perspectives on the use of grammaticality judgment tasks in linguistic theory. *Second Language Studies, 24*, 129–167. Retrieved from https://scholarspace.manoa.hawaii.edu/handle/10125/40679?mode=full

Tremblay, A. (2006). On the second language acquisition of Spanish reflexive passives and reflexive impersonals by French-and English-speaking adults. *Second Language Research, 22*, 30–63. https://doi.org/10.1191/0267658306sr260oa

Tuninetti, A., Warren, T., & Tokowicz, N. (2015). Cue strength in second-language processing: An eye-tracking study. *The Quarterly Journal of Experimental Psychology, 68*, 568–584.

Ullman, M.T. (2001). The neural basis of lexicon and grammar in first and second language: The declarative/procedural model. *Bilingualism: Language and Cognition, 4*, 105–122. https://doi.org/10.1017/S1366728901000220

Uziel, S. (1993). Resetting universal grammar parameters: Evidence from second language acquisition of subjacency and the empty category principle. *Second Language Research, 9*, 49–83. https://doi.org/10.1177/026765839300900103

Vafaee, P., Suzuki, Y., & Kachisnke, I. (2017). Validating grammaticality judgment tests: Evidence from two new psycholinguistic measures. *Studies in Second Language Acquisition, 39*, 59–95. https://doi.org/10.1017/S0272263115000455

Valenzuela, E., Faure, A., Ramírez-Trujillo, A. P., Barski, E., Pangtay, Y., & Diez, A. (2012). Gender and heritage Spanish bilingual grammars: A study of code-mixed determiner phrases and copula constructions. *Hispania, 95*, 481–494. https://doi.org/10.2307/23266150

VanPatten, B. (2012). Input processing. In S. Gass & A. Mackey (Eds.), *The Routledge handbook of second language acquisition* (pp. 268–281). New York, NY: Routledge.

VanPatten, B., & Williams, J. (2015). *Theories in second language acquisition: An introduction* (2nd ed.). New York, NY: Routledge.

Vygotsky, L. S. (1967). *Thought and language*. Cambridge, MA: MIT Press.

Vygotsky, L. S. (1978). *Mind in society: The development of higher psychological processes*. Cambridge, MA: Harvard University Press.

Wakabayashi, S. (1996). The nature of interlanguage: SLA of reflexives. *Second Language Research, 12*, 266–303. https://doi.org/10.1177/026765839601200302

Wartenburger, I., Heekeren, H. R., Abutalebi, J., Cappa, S. F., Villringer, A., & Perani, D. (2003). Early setting of grammatical processing in the bilingual brain. *Neuron, 37*, 159–170. https://doi.org/10.1016/S0896-6273(02)01150-9

Wasow, T., & Arnold, J. (2005). Intuitions in linguistic argumentation. *Lingua, 115*, 1481–1496. https://doi.org/10.1016/j.lingua.2004.07.001

Weber-Fox, C. M., & Neville, H. J. (1996). Maturational constraints on functional specializations for language processing: ERP and behavioral evidence in bilingual speakers. *Journal of Cognitive Neuroscience, 8*, 231–256.

Weskott, T., & Fanselow, G. (2011). On the informativity of different measures of linguistic acceptability. *Language, 87*, 249–273. https://doi.org/10.1353/lan.2011.0041

White, L. (1987). Markedness and second language acquisition: The question of transfer. *Studies in Second Language Acquisition, 9*, 261–286.

White, L. (1989). The adjacency condition on case assignment: Do L2 learners observe the Subset Principle? In S. Gass & J. Schachter (Eds.), *Linguistic perspectives on second language acquisition* (pp. 134–158). Cambridge: Cambridge University Press.

White, L. (1991). Adverb placement in second language acquisition: Some effects of positive and negative evidence in the classroom. *Interlanguage Studies Bulletin*, 7, 133–161.

White, L., Belikova, A., Hagstrom, P., Kupisch, T., & Özçelik, Ö. (2012). Restrictions on definiteness in second language acquisition: Affirmative and negative existentials in the L2 English of Turkish and Russian speakers. *Linguistic Approaches to Bilingualism, 2*, 56–84. https://doi.org/10.1075/lab.2.1.03whi

White, L., Bruhn-Garavito, J., Kawasaki, T., Pater, J., & Prévost, P. (1997). The researcher gave the subject a test about himself: Problems of ambiguity and preference in the investigation of reflexive binding. *Language Learning, 47*, 145–172. https://doi.org/10.1111/0023-8333.41997004

White, L., & Juffs, A. (1998). Constraints on wh-movement in two different contexts of non-native language acquisition: Competence and processing. In S. Flynn, G. Martohardjono, & W. O'Neill (Eds.), *The generative study of second language acquisition* (pp. 111–130) Hillsdale, NJ: Lawrence Erlbaum Associates.

White, J., & Ranta, L. (2002). Examining the interface between metalinguistic task performance and oral production in a second language. *Language Awareness, 11*, 259–290. https://doi.org/10.1080/09658410208667060

Winke, P. (2014). Testing hypotheses about language learning using structural equation modeling. *Annual Review of Applied Linguistics, 34*, 102–122. https://doi.org/10.1017/S0267190514000075

Yalçin, S., & Spada, N. (2016). Language aptitude and grammatical difficulty: An EFL classroom-based study. *Studies in Second Language Acquisition, 38*, 239–263. https://doi.org/10.1017/S0272263115000509

Yan, X., Maeda, Y., Lv, J., & Ginther, A. (2016). Elicited imitation as a measure of second language proficiency: A narrative review and meta-analysis. *Language Testing, 33*, 497–528. https://doi.org/10.1177/0265532215594643

Yang, J., & Li, P. (2012). Brain networks of explicit and implicit learning. *PLoS One*, 7. https://doi.org/10.1371/journal.pone.0042993

Yuan, B. (1995). Acquisition of base-generated topics by English-speaking learners of Chinese. *Language Learning, 45*, 567–603. https://doi.org/10.1111/j.1467-1770.1995.tb00455.x

Zaykovskaya, I. (in progress). *Perceptions of remarkable US English LIKE by native and non-native English-speaking young adults in Michigan* (Ph.D. dissertation), Michigan State University, East Lansing.

Zhang, D. (2012). Vocabulary and grammar knowledge in second language reading comprehension: A structural equation modeling study. *The Modern Language Journal, 96*, 558–575. https://doi.org/10.1111/j.1540-4781.2012.01398.x

Zhang, R. (2015). Measuring university-level L2 learners' implicit and explicit linguistic knowledge. *Studies in Second Language Acquisition, 37*, 457–486. https://doi.org/10.1017/S0272263114000370

Ziętek, A., & Roehr, K. (2011). Metalinguistic knowledge and cognitive style in Polish classroom learners of English. *System, 39*, 417–426. https://doi.org/10.1016/j.system.2011.05.005

Zufferey, S., Mak, W., Degand, L., & Sanders, T. (2015). Advanced learners' comprehension of discourse connectives: The role of L1 transfer across on-line and off-line tasks. *Second Language Research, 31*, 369–411. https://doi.org/10.1177/0267658315573349

Zydatiß, W. (1972). *Aspects of the language of German learners of English in the area of thematization* (Doctoral thesis), University of Edinburgh, Scotland.

INDEX

Note: Page numbers in *italics* indicate figures, and page numbers in **bold** indicate tables.